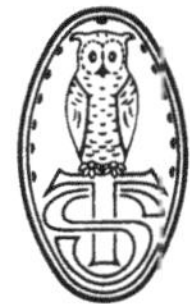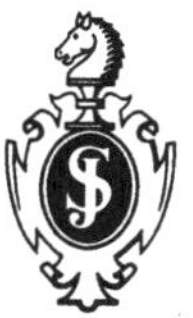

PTCA-Workshop
Munich, Germany
September 16–18, 1985

B. Höfling (Ed.)

Current Problems in PTCA

With Contributions by
T. von Arnim   U. W. Busch   J. S. Douglas Jr   R. Erbel
R. von Essen   E. Fleck   T. Ischinger   C.-M. Kirsch   G. Kober
H. C. Mehmel   B. Meier   B. Reichart   H. Riess   W. Rutsch
P. W. Serruys   R. Simon   M. A. J. Weber

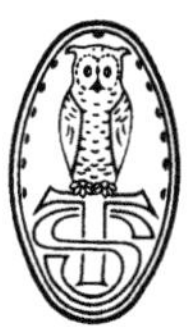

Steinkopff Verlag Darmstadt
Springer-Verlag New York

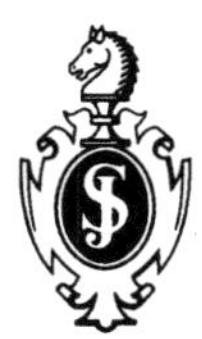

PD Dr. B. Höfling
Medizinische Klinik I
Klinikum Großhadern
Marchioninistraße 15
8000 München 70

CIP-Kurztitelaufnahme der Deutschen Bibliothek

Current problems in PTCA

[PTCA Workshop, Munich Germany September 16–18, 1985].
B. Höfling (ed.). With contributions by T. von Arnim . . .
Darmstadt: Steinkopff; New York: Springer, 1987.
ISBN-13:978-3-642-72409-1   e-ISBN-13:978-3-642-72407-7
DOI: 10.1007/978-3-642-72407-7

NE: Höfling, Berthold [Hrsg.]; Arnim, Thomas von [Mitverf.];
PTCA Workshop <1985, München>

Preface

Since coronary angioplasty was first practiced by Andreas Grüntzig in 1977, it has rapidly developed into a technique widely used on patients with chronic and acute coronary heart disease.

The meeting described in this book was held under the auspices of the working group of our national society, chaired by Prof. Kaltenbach, Frankfurt, and by Prof. Meyer, Mainz, in cooperation with Stanford University. It is an attempt to present various cardiologists' appraisals of the current position of PTCA in clinical medicine.

PTCA is far from easy, as its mechanism is critically balanced between success and failure. Therefore the experience of more than one hundred cases is generally regarded as necessary for cutting down complications and achieving a high rate of success. Furthermore, success *and* complications are a result not only of technical expertise, but also of patient selection.

The emphasis of the workshop was on discussion of some unsolved problems and open questions such as:

- What are the reliable indication guide-lines?
- What are the established guide-lines for deciding, once a complication occurs, between operative and non-operative treatment?
- What are the indications and limitations for the combined use of thrombolysis with PTCA in acute myocardial infarction?
- When and at what intervals should PTCA be applied after successful lysis?
- Who are the candidates for dilatation of mainstem stenosis?
- When should one attempt to open occluded arteries and which technique shows the most promise?
- Can we achieve from all our analyses a better and more creative understanding of the atherosclerotic process?

Finally, a word of thanks to all participants of the workshop, particularly to Dr. Höfling to whom J am greatly indebted. He brought together many cardiologists: those who usually select patients for PTCA without being directly involved in its practice, and those who strive to improve the patient's condition by application of dilatation techniques.

We are aware that our learning curve is still in ascendence and therefore fully appreciate the generosity of our most experienced colleagues in passing on their precious expertise through this book. We hope, then, that it will be of value to cardiologists in clinical medicine.

G. Riecker, Munich

Contents

Diagnostic Procedures Before, During, and After PTCA

B. Meier

Center for Cardiology, University Hospital, Geneva, Switzerland

Diagnostic Procedures for Indication of PTCA

Coronary Angiography

Before a patient is accepted for a diagnostic test, he or she should be screened for suitability to undergo therapeutic procedures that may ensue from it. If this rule is observed, the majority of patients undergoing coronary angiography already meet the clinical criteria for eligibility for PTCA in terms of age, angina pectoris, positive exercise test, and absence of concomitant life-threatening disease.

Coronary angiography is not only the gold standard for assessing the degree of disease but also the backbone of therapeutic planning. On the basis of a coronary angiogram, patients with similar clinical pictures may be declared healthy, shown to have vasospastic angina, treated medically for nonsignificant disease, referred for urgent bypass surgery for menacing triple-vessel disease, considered inoperable, or accepted for PTCA. The criteria to opt for surgical therapy, medical therapy, or PTCA may vary with time and from operator to operator, but they are primarily based on angiographic findings.

Other Diagnostic Tests

In borderline cases, an exercise test may indicate when to intervene, a thallium-201 study may identify a myocardial region thought to be ischemic as already infarcted, or certain findings of the left ventriculogram may dictate an operation although the coronary anatomy would be suitable for PTCA. These auxiliary tests, however, are more important for the assessment of initial and late results than for the indication of PTCA.

Assessment of Results

The result of PTCA can be subdivided into the in-laboratory result, the in-hospital result, and the long-term result.

In-Laboratory-Result

There are several means of monitoring the result of PTCA during the procedure itself. They are, in order of accuracy and helpfulness: pressure gradient, angiography, electrocardiogram, systemic blood pressure, and coronary flow measurement. More subjective but nonetheless helpful are the symptoms reported by the patient.

Pressure Gradient. The trans-stenotic pressure gradient may not be available with certain types of dilatation catheters or in situations where the guiding catheter completely obstructs the coronary orifice. It may be artificially high if the vessel lumen is small compared with the size of the deflated balloon [1].

This typically is the case when the initial gradient of a tight stenosis is measured (overestimated initial pressure gradient) or with PTCA in small vessels (overestimated initial and residual pressure gradient). A low or abolished residual pressure gradient after PTCA, however, is reliable, and is the most important indicator of a favorable hemodynamic result of the intervention. There is no such thing as a falsely low residual pressure gradient, provided that the pressure systems are properly calibrated and checked for leaks.

The pressure gradient guides throughout the procedures. Initially, it corroborates the indication for PTCA. (A stenosis with an initial gradient of < 20 mmHg should not be dilated unless the gradient increase with hyperemia is induced by a drug, exercise, or cardiac pacing.) After each balloon filling, the pressure gradient indicates the intermediate result and the need for further dilatation maneuvers or balloon exchanges. About 30 s should be allowed for the postocclusion hyperemia to settle [2]. The final gradient accepted as satisfactory is arbitrary. It is rarely affected by additional vasodilators if they have been administered prophylactically at the beginning of the procedure. If two consecutive balloon fillings for at least 1 min with adequate balloon size and pressure fail to improve the residual pressure gradient to < 20 mmHg, an unfavorable position of the intimal flap created by PTCA usually has to be assumed. The angiographic result may still be acceptable, but there is a higher chance of recurrence [3]. The average initial and final pressure gradients of a large series of patients were 48 and 12 mmHg respectively [4].

The assessment of the coronary wedge pressure (pressure distal to the stenosis during balloon occlusion) makes it possible to determine the degree of collateralization of the dilated vessel [5]. This measurement should be performed after at least 30 s of occlusion and at low balloon pressure, e.g., 2 bar. High balloon pressure may compress the pressure channel and reveal an artificially high coronary wedge pressure. The presence or absence of collaterals to the diseased vessel is of paramount importance for the immediate risk of the intervention and for the long-term risk of the patient. Collaterals are visible on a diagnostic coronary angiogram only if a subtotal stenosis is present. With a lesser stenosis, they may still be on standby and recruitable in the event of acute vessel occlusion [5]. A coronary wedge pressure of > 30 mmHg indicates the presence of collaterals.

Angiography. At least two (preferably perpendicular) projections are needed to accurately assess a coronary stenosis during PTCA. They are chosen from the initial angiogram or from several projections filmed immediately before PTCA.

After each balloon inflation, 0.5 ml of contrast medium is injected through the balloon catheter to observe the runoff. The briskness of the runoff provides qualitative hemodynamic information. Moreover, the tip of the balloon catheter is cleared of blood to prevent clogging and assure accurate pressure transmission.

After withdrawal of the balloon, with the coronary guide wire still across the stenosis, the angiographic result is checked with an injection through the guiding catheter. It is difficult to inject a sufficient amount of contrast medium through a guiding catheter contain-

2

ing a balloon catheter. Contrast medium delivery can be improved by using a small-caliber syringe or a power injector, by simultaneous injection through both guiding catheter and balloon catheter, or by completely withdrawing the balloon catheter from the guiding catheter. The latter technique requires a long coronary guide wire [6].

In any case, the final result will only be apparent once the guide wire has been retracted from the coronary artery and a decent contrast injection has been filmed and reviewed (preferably on cinefilm). Yet, an attempt to return to improve the result at this time may be detrimental, because the dissection created by the angioplasty may guide the wire into a false lumen and vessel occlusion may occur. Therefore, parameters other than fluoroscopy (pressure gradient, electrocardiogram, chest pain, etc.) should be exhausted to avoid the need of additional catheterization of a freshly dilated vessel.

If collaterals were present before angioplasty, a contralateral injection at the end of the intervention is of interest. Disappearance of the collaterals reflects a good hemodynamic result and can be predicted if the final pressure gradient has been measured. In case of multiple-vessel PTCA and presence of collaterals, the recipient vessel should be dilated first. The vessel providing the collaterals should be attempted only if the collateralization is no longer visible or is reversed in direction after completion of PTCA of the first vessel. If PTCA of the vessel providing the collaterals is performed first, two myocardial areas will be devoid of blood flow in the event of vessel obstruction. This subjects the patient to an unacceptable risk.

Electrocardiogram. Several ECG leads, or at least the lead best reflecting the myocardial area at risk, are to be monitored continuously throughout PTCA. Assistants and laboratory personnel should be trained and encouraged to keep an eye on the ECG and pressure monitor and to alert the operator to all relevant changes. Care should be taken not to alarm the patient. ST elevation after placement of the balloon catheter in a tight stenosis or during balloon fillings is normal but should be reversible within a few minutes. The coronary guide wire can be used as an additional intracoronary ECG lead (Fig. 1). It allows for extremely sensitive monitoring of ischemic changes of the pertinent myocardium [7]. Ectopic beats may be provoked by advancing the coronary guide wire into a small side-branch, e.g., a septal branch. They are therefore of help in correctly positioning the guide wire. Ectopic beats or bradycardia due to flow obstruction are ominous and require immediate reestablishment of flow, or antiarrhythmic therapy or cardiac pacing if flow cannot be restored.

Systemic Blood Pressure. Observation of the systemic blood pressure on the monitor helps one to react in time to drug-induced, vagovasal, or allergic hypotension, to hypertension due to anxiety of the patient, or to acute left heart failure due to ischemia. In addition, the systemic pressure measured through the guiding catheter drops if the catheter is advanced into wedging position. Although a low reading in such a setting does not reflect systemic hypotension, it reflects absence of coronary flow and should be remedied.

Coronary Flow. Assessment of coronary flow reserve provides an additional hemodynamic parameter. Special electronic equipment is required for this technique, based on comparison of contrast flow velocity in a coronary artery at rest and during induced hyperemia [8]. It may be useful during follow-up angiography when the trans-stenotic pressure gradient is not available.

Coronary vein flow measurements before, during and after PTCA revealed that resting flow in the great cardiac vein does not increase after successful PTCA of the left anterior descending coronary artery. Hyperemic flow, however, increases [2, 9].

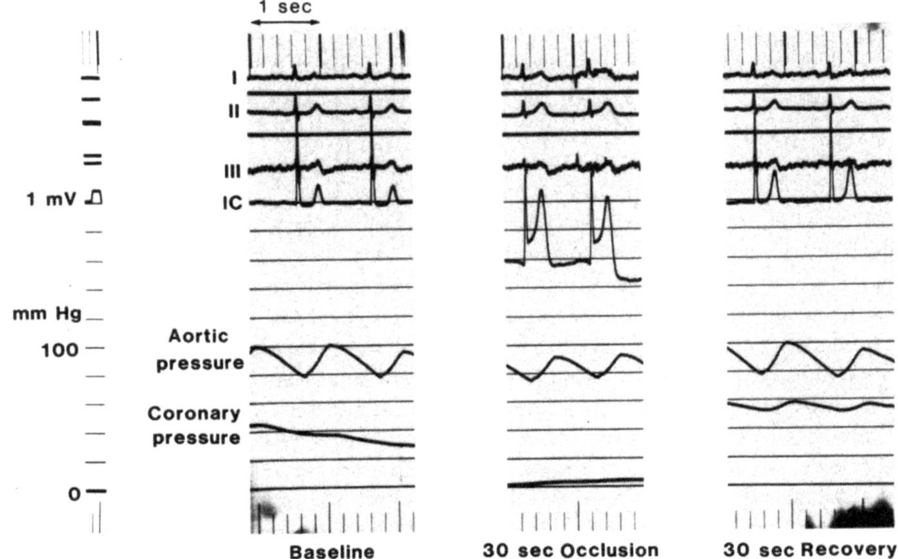

Fig. 1. Intracoronary ECG and pressure tracings during PTCA of the left circumflex coronary artery of a 50-year-old woman. The intracoronary (*IC*) lead show reversible 2-mV ST elevation during balloon occlusion, while the standard leads, I, II and III show only minimal changes

Patient's Complaints. Persistent mild chest pain for about an hour after uncomplicated PTCA is not an uncommon finding. Its origin remains to be determined. The pain may be secondary to intimal dissection with localized wall hemorrhage, commonly occurring with PTCA. Increasing chest pain after PTCA, however, needs to be investigated and will most commonly be reflected by ECG changes. Progressive vessel occlusion by spasm or dislocation of an intimal flap with or without concomitant thrombosis are likely causes. Continuous interrogation of the patient about chest pain during PTCA helps the operator to become aware of complications such as side branch occlusion or flow deterioration in a vessel dilated in the same session. These complications may not be recognizable otherwise.

The character of chest pain during balloon occlusion should be compared with the angina experienced at home. If it is identical, the operator may be assured that he or she is treating the source of the patient's problem.

In-Hospital Result

Patient interrogation, ECG, telemetry (if available), and creatine kinase levels are used for patient monitoring during the first 12 h after the intervention. After mobilization the functional result is assessed by a stress test.

Electrocardiogram. Two postinterventional ECGs should be compared with the preinterventional one, the first upon return from the catheterization laboratory and the second the next day (this may be combined with the stress test). Any chest pain refractory to

4

nitroglycerine and calcium antagonists should prompt an additional ECG. Signs of acute ischemia persisting for > 20 min call for immediate action, be it repeat PTCA, fibrinolysis, or emergency bypass surgery.

Creatine Kinase. Serial creatine kinase determination is not necessary with uncomplicated PTCA [10]. The value will slightly rise after PTCA but will stay within normal limits. In case of complications, however, the creatine kinase level should be assessed at regular intervals to estimate the amount of damage.

Functional Result

For the patient, functional improvement is the most important benefit from PTCA. An exercise test as a quantitative functional assessment should be performed in all cases, preferably before hospital discharge.

Bicycle ergometry after angiographically successful PTCA showed a marked increase in mean work capacity 2 days after the procedure [11]. Improvement of myocardial perfusion and myocardial function during exercise after PTCA was documented by a thallium-201 scan [12, 13] and nuclear assessment of ejection fraction [14]. Thallium-201 defects

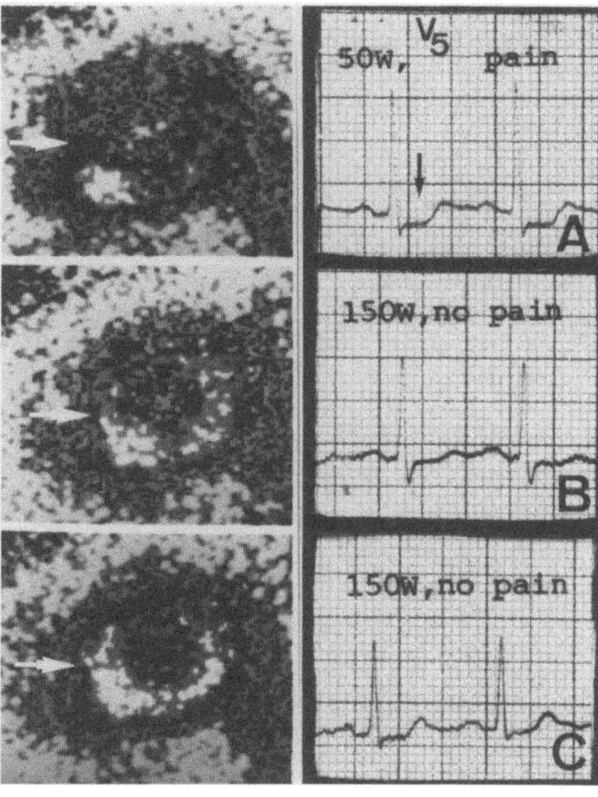

Fig. 2a-C. Thallium-201 stress test the day before (A), the day after (B), and 1 month after (C) PTCA of the proximal left anterior descending coronary artery in a 61-year-old man. The pictures were taken in a 70° left anterior oblique projection at peak exercise which was 50 W (heart rate 115/min) for A, 150 W (120/min) for B, and 150 W (112/min) for C. The test was clinically positive before and clinically negative after PTCA. There is reduced thallium-201 uptake in the myocardial area of concern (anteroseptal wall) in A as compared with B and C (*arrow*), and there is significant ST depression in A but not in B and C (lead V5)

disappear after successful PTCA, as do regional and global ejection fraction abnormalities determined by a nuclear scan during atrial pacing. Figure 2 shows normalization of a thallium-201 stress test with successful PTCA.

Long-Term Result

The assessment of long-term results is based on subjective findings and stress tests. Angiographic controls are important in special situations.

Subjective Findings

Patients are encouraged to be physically active and to return to work immediately after hospital discharge if the result of PTCA is satisfactory. Regular physical activity serves as a daily functional test to herald restenosis. If physical activity begins to be restricted by angina, a stress test should be performed and compared with the test done before and immediately after PTCA.

Stress Tests

In stable or asymptomatic patients stress tests seem appropriate after 3, 6, and 12 months and then annually. A normal stress test in patients who had an abnormal stress test before PTCA is a good indicator of sustained patency of the dilated vessel [15].

Control Angiography

If control angiography is not done routinely, it should be done in all patients with recurrent symptoms or deterioration of stress test performance as soon as these harbingers of restenosis appear. Control angiography in asymptomatic patients may corroborate the favorable impression gained by subjective findings and functional tests and allow for discontinuation of heart medication. If done about one year after PTCA, the chance of missing a later recurrence is remote [16].
The diagnosis of long-term success or recurrence, however, should not be based on an angiogram alone; it should be derived from a synopsis of angiogram, functional tests, and subjective complaints.

References

1. Leiboff R, Bren G, Katz R, Korkegi R, Ross A (1983) Determinants of trans-stenotic gradients observed during angioplasty: an experimental model. Am J Cardiol 52: 1311-1317
2. Rothman MT, Baim DS, Simpson JB, Harrison DC (1982) Coronary hemodynamics during percutaneous transluminal coronary angioplasty. Am J Cardiol 49: 1615-1622

3. Holmes DR jr, Vlietstra RE, Smith HC, Vetrovec GW, Kent KM, Cowley MJ, Faxon DP, Grüntzig AR, Kelsey SF, Detre KM, van Raden MJ, Mock MB (1984) Restenosis after percutaneous transluminal coronary angioplasty (PTCA): a report from the PTCA registry of the National Heart, Lung, and Blood Institute. Am J Cardiol 53: 77C-81C

4. Ischinger T, Grüntzig AR (1984) Perkutane transluminale Koronarangioplastie. In: Roskamm H (ed) Handbuch der inneren Medizin, vol IX, 3. Springer-Verlag, Berlin Heidelberg New York, pp 1301-1317

5. Meier B, Luethy P (1984) Coronary wedge pressure as predictor of recruitable coronary arteries (abstr.). Circulation 70 (II): II-266

6. Kaltenbach M (1985) The long-wire technique – a new technique for steerable balloon catheter dilatation of coronary artery stenoses. Eur Heart J 5: 1004-1009

7. Meier B, Killisch JP, Adatte JJ, Casalini P, Rutishauser W (1985) Intrakoronares EKG während transluminaler Koronarangiographie. Schweiz Med Wochenschr 155: 1590-1593

8. O'Neill WW, Walton JA, Bates ER, Colfer HT, Aueron FM, LeFree MT, Pitt D, Vogel RA (1984) Criteria for successful coronary angioplasty as assessed by alterations in coronary vasodilatory reserve. J Am Coll Cardiol 3: 1382-1390

9. Serruys PW, Wijns W, van den Brand M, Meij S, Slager C, Schuurbiers JCH, Hugenholtz PG, Brower RW (1984) Left ventricular performance, regional blood flow, wall motion, and lactate metabolism during transluminal angioplasty. Circulation 70: 25-36

10. Berclaz S, Meier B, Barthélémy JC, Rutishauser W (1985) Changes in creatine phosphokinase after coronary angioplasty. In: Meyer J, Erbel R, Rupprecht HJ (eds) Improvement of myocardial perfusion – thrombolysis, angioplasty, bypass surgery. Martinus Nijhoff, Boston, pp 201-203

11. Meier B, Grüntzig AR, Siegenthaler WE, Schlumpf M (1983) Long-term exercise performance after percutaneous transluminal coronary angioplasty and coronary artery bypass grafting. Circulation 68: 796-802

12. Kanemoto N, Hör G, Kober G, Maul FD, Klepzig H Jr, Standke R, Kaltenbach M (1983) Non-invasive assessment of left ventricular performance following transluminal coronary angioplasty Int. J Cardiol 3: 281-292

13. Hirzel HO, Nuesch K, Grüntzig AR, Luetolf UM (1981) Short- and long-term changes in myocardial perfusion after percutaneous transluminal coronary angioplasty assessed by thallium-201 exercise scintigraphy. Circulation 63: 1001-1007

14. Weiss AT, Gotsman MS, Shefer A, Halon DA, Lewis BS (1984) Improvement in regional ventricular function after percutaneous transluminal coronary angioplasty. Int J Cardiol 5: 299-311

15. Scholl JM, Chaitman BR, David PR, Dupras G, Brévers G, Val PG, Crépeau J, Lespérance J, Bourassa MG (1982) Exercise electrocardiography and myocardial scintigraphy in the serial evaluation of the results of percutaneous transluminal coronary angioplasty. Circulation 66: 380-389

16. Meier B, King SB III, Grüntzig AR, Douglas JS, Hollman J, Ischinger T, Galan K, Tankersley R (1984) Repeat coronary angioplasty. J Am Coll Cardiol 4: 463-466

Author's address:
Dr. Bernhard Meier
Centre de Cardiologie
Hôpital Cantonal Universitaire
CH-1211 Genève 4
Switzerland

Current Indications for PTCA

B. Höfling[1], T. von Arnim[1], A. Stäblein[1], E. Kreuzer[2], and B. Kemkes[2]

[1] Medical Dept. I, Klinikum Großhadern, University of Munich
[2] Heart Surgery Dept., Klinikum Großhadern, University of Munich

Introduction

The primary indications for PTCA have changed considerably in the past few years and
continue to expand. There are two major reasons for this development. One is that improved equipment and technology favor new and additional approaches. In particular,
the advanced X-ray generation enables the investigator to visualize the lesion optimally
and to control the procedure better, with a consequent decrease in risk, complications, or
failure. Also, fluoroscopy time and the amount of contrast medium can be reduced. Furthermore, the balloon catheter design has been fundamentally changed. John Simpson
was the first to develop and apply the independently movable intracoronary (i.c.) guide
wire [15, 32, 33]. There is a consensus that the primary success rate increased from 60%
to 80% or 90% after introduction of the i.c. guide wire.
The second reason for additional PTCA indications is the advanced experience and skill
of cardiologists performing angioplasty. Between established PTCA teams the technical
standard varies considerably, and it is widely accepted that even rather competent teams
should have experts available to whom difficult patients can be referred.
Consequently, not only are the indications themselves a very debatable issue; the indication criteria cover a wide range depending on the experience of the respective cardiologist.

Clinical Indications

Clinical indications for balloon dilatation are (Fig. 1):
- Anginal symptoms which are refractory to medical management
- Objective evidence of myocardial ischemia by means of a stress test or radionuclide in-
  vestigation

If a high-grade stenosis is combined with angina pectoris class III or IV in spite of therapy, angioplasty is indicated if the lesion can be approached by PTCA (Fig. 1a). Stress
tests and thallium scintigraphy are of minor importance in these patients.
A more difficult group are the relatively asymptomatic patients who have a high-grade
stenosis which might be correlated to an inherent extensive infarction. Since symptoms
are not severe, this intervention could be regarded as prophylactic. In general, we hold
the conception that any prophylactic intervention is a possibly dangerous action. Therefore, with these patients we follow the guidelines which were defined by the National

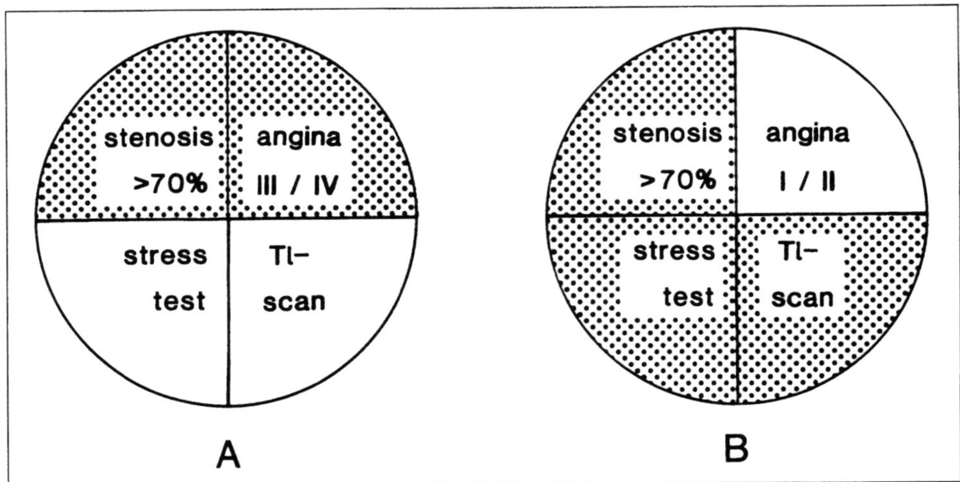

Fig. 1a,b. Clinical indications for PTCA in patients with (**a**) and without (**b**) symptoms of angina

Council on Scientific Affairs (NCSA) in 1982 and published in 1984 [4]: PTCA is indicated if there is "strong objective evidence of myocardial ischemia" from one or two objective investigations (Fig. 1b). Results of thallium scintigraphy and stress tests have a major impact on decision-making in this group of patients.

Angiographic Indications

From the angiographic standpoint (Table 1), the indications are not as clear as those based on clinical characteristics. The indication list should be individualized for each angioplasty group.

The easiest stenosis to treat is that coming closest to the "ideal stenosis". However, it must be pointed out that attempted or even successful PTCA of a so-called ideal stenosis may also result in an occlusion, with subsequent myocardial infarction or death. This is due to the mechanism of PTCA, which is not compression of the atheroma as was initially assumed. Experimental investigations and pathological examinations have shown that plaque rupture and splitting of intima and media with local dissection are inevitable and must be regarded as part of the mechanism of successful PTCA [1, 17, 26, 35]. A primary successful PTCA may also be followed by subendothelial hematomas [36]. These mechanisms may cause acute vessel occlusions even several hours after termination of an initially perfect procedure.

The published figures for primary success, complications, and death refer to a patient population with more than 75% "ideal stenoses" [7, 28]. These figures improve with growing experience, but they deteriorate with extended and risky indications even in advanced groups. A balance has been created between increasing experience and introduction of new indications.

Table 1. Angiographic indications for PTCA

Extended clinical indications	
	− unstable angina pectoris
	− myocardial infarction
„Ideal" stenoses	New indications
− single-vessel disease	− distal lesion
− proximal	− eccentric
− concentric	− calcified
− noncalcified	− serial stenoses
− short	− occluded vessels
− straight	− multivessel disease
− no side branches	− impaired LV function
− good collaterals	− bypass lesion
	− intraoperative, combined procedure
	− repeat angioplasty
	− elderly patients
	− not suitable for ACBS
	− lesion in minor vessels

In Table 1 the angiographic indications for PTCA are summarized, beginning with a desscription of the "ideal stenosis". The extension to the other types of coronary lesions can be realized stepwise, with increasing expertise and willingness to extend the application to patients at risk. It has even been stated that "[today] there is no general contraindication for PTCA" [30].

Some important examples of "new indications" should be mentioned in particular:

− For *distal lesions* (Fig. 2): The independently movable i.c. guide wire was the prerequisite for finding and reaching distal lesions with low risk before following with the balloon. One difficulty is that, when passing curves, the "back power" needed for pushing the balloon into tight stenoses may be lost, even if the guiding catheter has a stable position at the ostium. Sometimes soft guiding catheters can be advanced far down into the vessel to regain "back power".

− There is no dispute about the fact that *eccentric lesions* can be approached. Statistical analyses have shown that risk and primary success with eccentric lesions are in the same range as with concentric lesions, or slightly elevated [3].

− Today, *calcification* is not considered to be a contraindication for PTCA. However, in our experience, and according to reports of others, the primary success is decreased and the risk of complicating dissection is increased in this situation [3].

− For the assessment of *serial stenoses* an insignificantly lower primary success rate must be taken into account.

− *Impaired left ventricular function* can be regarded from two points of view. The risk of severe complications might be expected to increase if vessel occlusion occurs with concomitant additional decrease of left ventricular performance. On the other hand, we have had cases with remarkable improvement of left ventricular function after PTCA [Fig. 3]. We therefore conclude that, although PTCA risk may be increased in patients

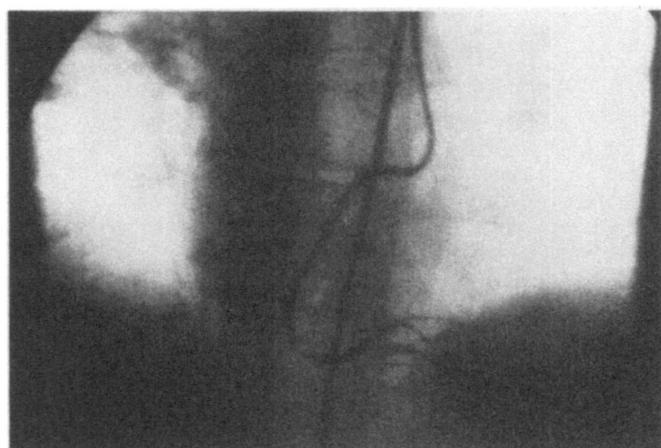

pre PTCA

Fig. 2. Distal lesion in a right coronary artery. Although the lesion is far from the ostium, it can easily be reached and crossed by the intracoronary wire. The balloon is then guided by the stable wire and is inflated after having been placed adequately

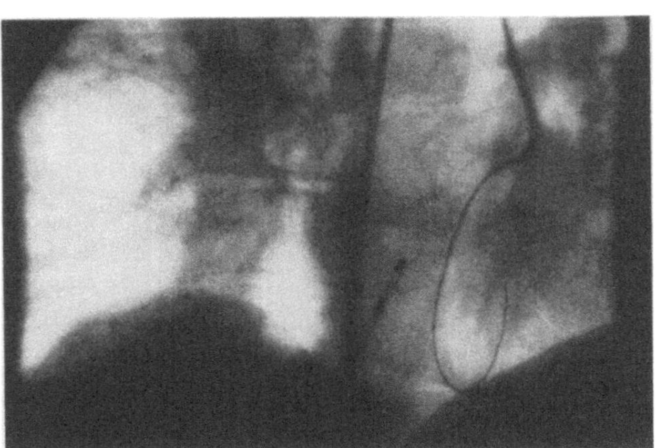

balloon in position

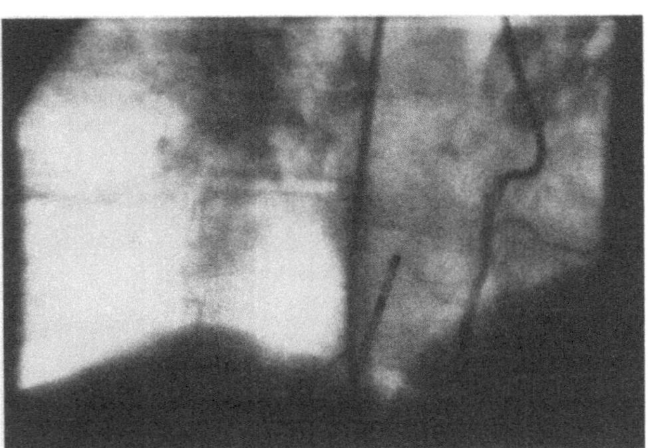

post PTCA

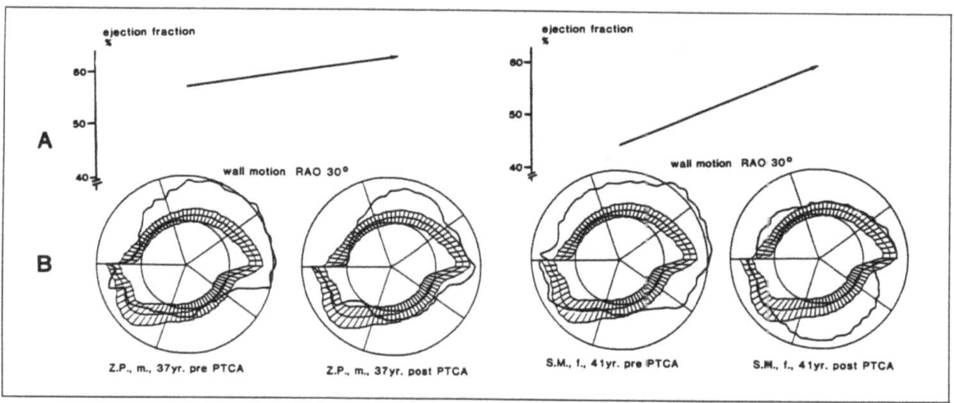

Fig. 3 Improvement of global (**A**) and regional (**B**) LV function after PTCA in two selected cases

with impaired left ventricular function, dilatation can be especially beneficial in selected cases with regional contraction deficit.

- One effective additional indication for PTCA is the approach to *occluded vessels* (Fig. 4). If the occlusion is recent and the occluded segment short, the probability of reopening the vessel is high [18, 20, 31]. However, after an occlusion of 2 months or longer the rate of early success falls to about 50%, with a reocclusion rate of 50% after successful recanalization. Consequently, the long-term success is only 25% [21]. These figures emphasize the fact that recanalization should be achieved early, if possible within the first 3 h after occlusion.
- PTCA has taken on an important role in the treatment of *acute myocardial infarction* [6, 14, 24]. This issue is thoroughly covered in the article by Rutsch et al., this volume.
- Balloon dilatation is also a well-established method for treating *unstable angina*: Meyer et al. [25] have convincingly demonstrated that PTCA is as effective in unstable angina as in stable angina [12].
- The extension of PTCA from single-vessel disease to *multivessel disease* is a major issue [5, 8, 16]. Certainly, the risk increases with the number of stenoses approached, independent of the operator's experience. But it appears that gifted angioplasty operators may treat patients with multivessel disease as effectively as bypass surgeons do.
- *Bypass stenoses* (Fig. 5) can be especially attractive for PTCA, since reoperation is more difficult and carries a fourfold mortality. PTCA in previously operated patients is connected with several disadvantages, however:
1. The coronary heart disease is often in an advanced state.
2. The patency rate after successful PTCA of bypass vessels is only around 50%, compared with 70% or 80% in native vessels.
3. In cases of acute occlusion the emergency operation is difficult and time consuming. Consequently, it is not surprising that analysis of lethal events during PTCA shows that a major determinant for mortality is a pre-existing bypass operation [2, 9, 10].
- *Intraoperative dilatation,* especially of distal lesions, could be expected to be a promising tool, but, after initial attempts, we feel that the digital control of the balloon cathe-

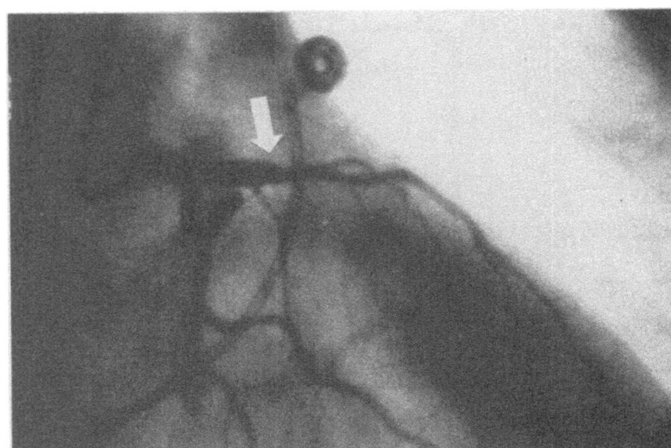

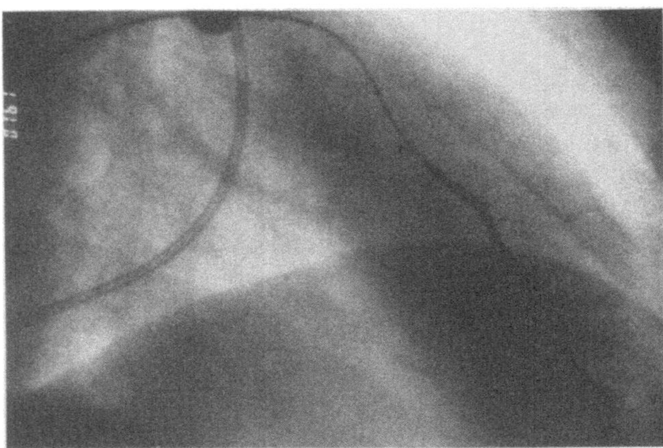

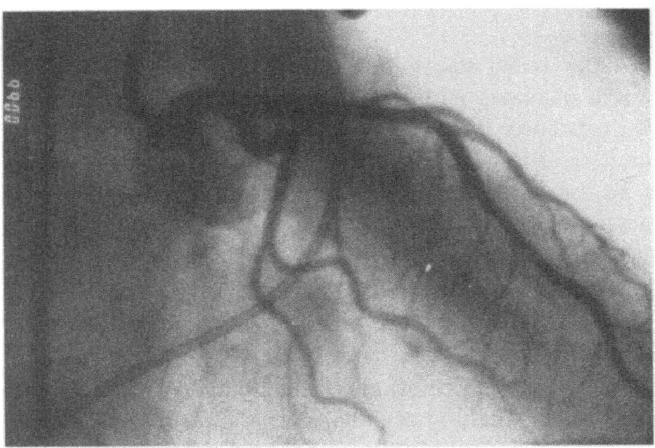

Fig. 4a-c. Successful PTCA of an occluded vessel. **a** Pre PTCA (occluded LAD after the first diagonal branch). **b** Distal contrast injection after the occlusion has been crossed with wire and ballon. **c** Post PTCA (recanalized LAD with numerous side branches)

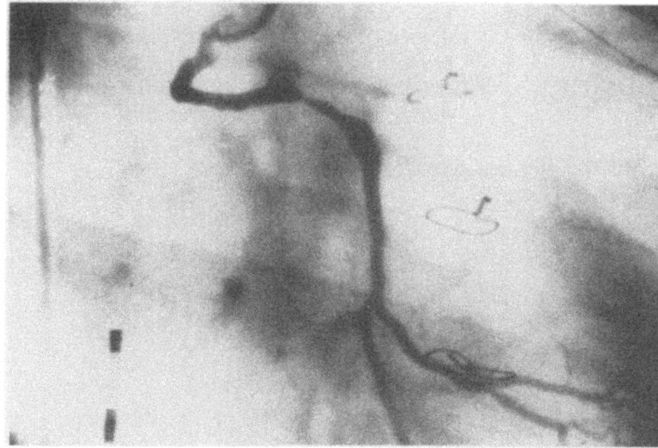

Fig. 5. PTCA of a bypass stenosis

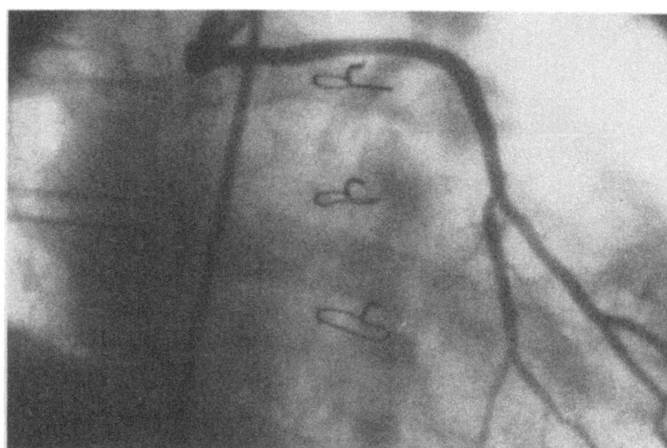

ter in small collapsed vessels of the asystolic heart is insufficient. We are not surprised that the reports in the literature [11, 13, 19] refer to small numbers, and the success rate is not convincing. It is worth considering whether the theoretically promising approach can be optimized by complementary PTCA during or after the end of the bypass operation under common fluoroscopic control with the established technique.

– Concerning *repeat angioplasty* of restenoses, it is generally accepted that the second intervention is technically easier and as effective as the first; it increases the long-term patency rate for the individual vessel from 70%, acquired with the first dilatation, to 90%, acquired with the second [22].

– Certain *elderly patients* may benefit from PTCA, although advanced age inevitably increases the risk [27, 29].

– In patients *unsuitable for bypass surgery*, PTCA may offer an alternative. For example, operation was hardly possible in the cases shown in Fig. 6, where the surgeons did not expect to find graft vessels after long periods of varicosis or dialysis.

– We have also learned that the dilatation of stenoses in small *side branches* can bring surprising relief of severe chest pain.

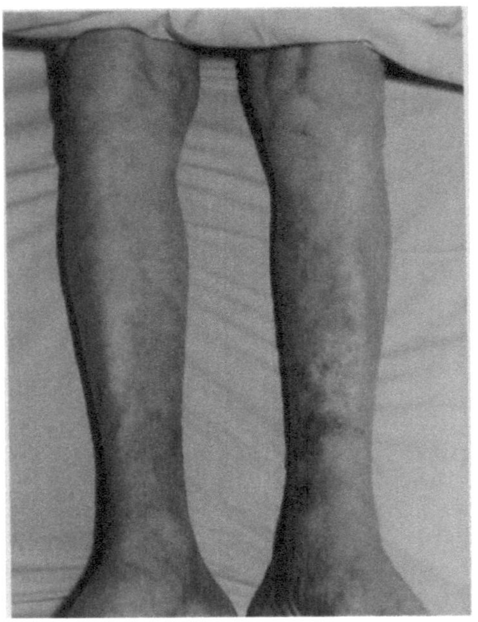

Fig. 6a–c. Two patients with coronary heart disease presenting foreseeable difficulties in the harvesting of bypass vessels. **a** Long history of varicosis, **b,c** 15-year history of dialysis with multiple shunts on all extremities

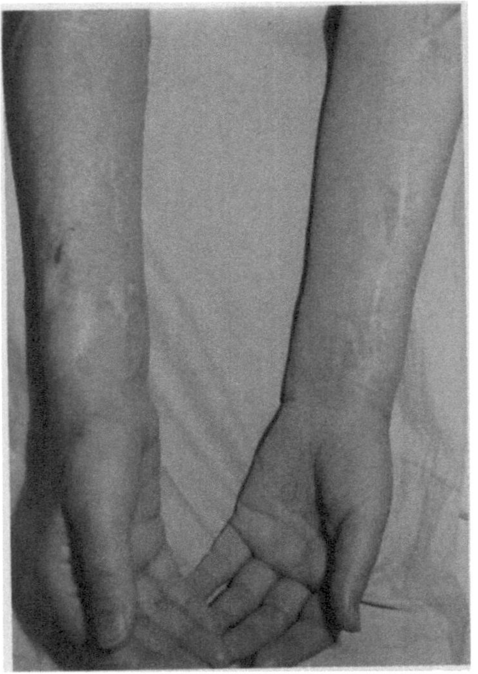

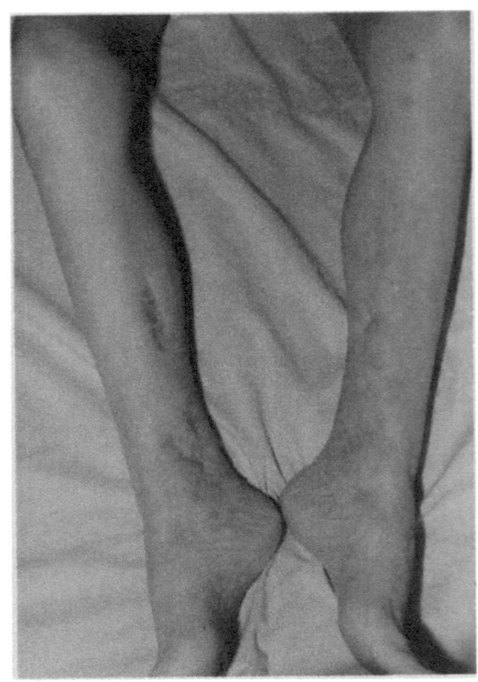

- If *coronary spasm* occurs during PTCA and cannot be relieved by drugs, a dilatation may be recommended; this is mostly effective in combination with i.c. administration of nitroglycerine or nifedipine. In contrast, if a *vasospastic angina* is identified before attempted PTCA, then medical treatment is the first choice and surgery the next option.
- The *length of the lesion* is not as important as was thought some years ago. But even today, PTCA is not recommended for lesions which are longer than 2 cm.

Borderline Cases and Containdications

Often, *major branching* is also not suitable for PTCA. This situation is dangerous because PTCA could occlude a major branch. Therefore, the NCSA allocates major branching to contraindications [4]. Even when acute occlusion of one vessel during dilatation in the

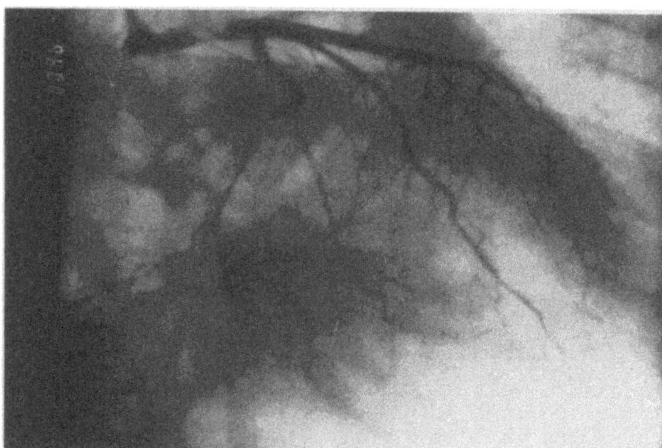

Fig. 7. Main-stem dilatation in a patient with foreseeable lack of bypass vessels (same patient as in Fig. 6a)

pre PTCA

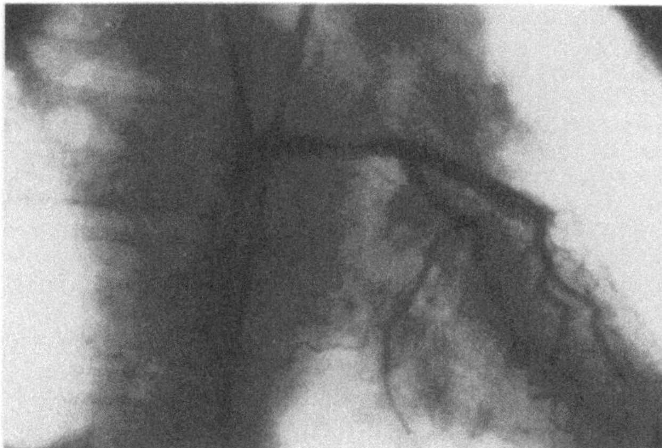

post PTCA

other can be prevented with the "kissing balloon" technique [23], we believe that a sequential bypass is the superior approach.

Caution should be exercised when dilating a *dominant vessel, since local occlusion with major infarction may quickly lead to shock. It has been known for many years that Killip class-IV infarctions have a lethal outcome in up to 90% of cases. In this situation, reperfusion catheters may help to stabilize the patient until bypass surgery brings relief.*

We feel that *main stem stenoses* are usually a contraindication, because death is most likely if the vessel occludes during or after PTCA. Though we accept this as a basic rule, we now and then make an exception, as have other groups [34]. Figure 7 illustrates successful dilatation in a 52-year-old man, performed in the operating theatre after he had been anesthetized and cannulated in the groin.

References

1. Block PC, Myler RK, Stertzer S, Fallon T (1981) Morphology after transluminal angioplasty in human beings. N Engl J Med 305 (7): 382
2. Block PC, Cowley MJ, Kaltenbach M, Kent KM, Simpson JB (1984) Percutaneous angioplasty of bypass grafts or of bypass graft anastomotic sites. Am J Cardiol 53: 666
3. Bredlau CE, Roubin GS, Leimgruber PP, Douglas JS, King SB, Grüntzig AR (1984) In-hospital morbidity and mortality in patients undergoing elective coronary angioplasty. Circulation 72: 1044
4. Council on Scientific Affairs (1984) Percutaneous transluminal angioplasty. JAMA 251: 764
5. Cowley MJ, Vetrovec GW, DiSciasco G, Lewis SA, Hirsh PD, Wolfgang TC (1985) Coronary angioplasty of multiple vessels: short-term outcome and long-term results. Circulation 72: 1314
6. Dodge HT, Sheehan FH, Mathey DG, Brown BG, Kennedy JW (1985) Usefulness of coronary artery bypass graft surgery or percutaneous transluminal angioplasty after thrombolytic therapy. Circulation 72 [Suppl V]: V39
7. Dorros G, Cowley MJ, Simpson J, Bentivoglio LG, Block PC, Bourassa M, Detre K, Gosselin AJ, Grüntzig AR, Kelsey SF, Kent KM, Mock MB, Mullin SM, Myler RK, Passamani ER, Stertzer SH, Williams DO (1983) Percutaneous transluminal coronary angioplasty: report of complications from the National Heart, Lung and Blood Institute PTCA Registry. Circulation 67: 723
8. Dorros G, Stertzer SH, Cowley MJ, Myler RK (1984) Complex coronary angioplasty: multiple coronary dilatations. Am J Cardiol 53 [Suppl]:126C
9. Dorros G, Johnson WD, Tector AJ, Schmahl TM, Kalush SL, Janke L (1984) Percutaneous transluminal coronary angioplasty in patients with prior coronary artery bypass grafting. J Thorac Cardiovasc Surg 87: 17
10. Douglas JS, Grüntzig AR, King SB, Hollman J, Ischinger T, Meier B, Craver JM, Jones EL, Waller JL, Bone DK, Guyton R (1983) Percutaneous transluminal coronary angioplasty in patients with prior coronary bypass surgery. Am Coll Cardiol 2: 745
11. Faro RS, Alexander JA, Feldman RL, Pepine CJ, Conti CR, Knauf DG, Roberts AJ (1984) Intraoperative balloon-catheter dilatation: University of Florida experience. Am Heart J 107: 841
12. Faxon DP, Detre KM, McCabe CH, Fisher L, Holmes DR, Cowley MJ, Bourassa MG, van Raden M, Ryan TJ (1984) Role of percutaneous transluminal coronary angioplasty in the treatment of unstable angina: report from the National Heart, Lung and Blood Institute percutaneous transluminal coronary angioplasty and coronary artery study registries. Am J Cardiol 53 [Suppl]: 131C
13. Fogarty TJ, Kinney TB (1984) Intraoperative coronary artery balloon-catheter dilatation. Am Heart J 107: 845
14. Gold HK, Cowley MJ, Palacios IF, Vetrovec GW, Atkins CW, Block PC, Leinbach RC (1984) Combined intracoronary streptokinase infusion and coronary angioplasty during acute myocardial infarction Am J Cardiol 53 [Suppl]: 122C

15. Grüntzig AR, Hollman J (1982) Improved primary success rate in transluminal coronary angioplasty using a steerable guidance system. Circulation 66: 330
16. Hartzler GO (1985) Complex coronary angioplasty: an alternative therapy. Int J Cardiol 9: 133
17. Holmes DR, Vlietstra RE, Mock MB, Reeder GS, Smith HC, Bove AA, Bresnahan JF, Piehler JM, Schaff HV, Orszulak TA (1983) Angiographic changes produced by percutaneous transluminal coronary angioplasty. Am J Cardiol 51: 676
18. Holmes DR, Vlietstra RE (1985) Angioplasty in total coronary arterial occlusion. Herz 10: 292
19. Jones EJ, King SB (1984) Intraoperative balloon-catheter dilatation in the treatment of coronary artery disease. Am Heart J 107: 836
20. Kereiakes DJ, Selmon MR, McAuley BJ, McAuley DB, Sheehan DJ, Simpson JB (1985) Angioplasty in total coronary artery occlusion: experience in 76 consecutive patients. J Am Coll Cardiol 6: 526
21. Kober G, Hopf R, Reinemer H, Kaltenbach M (1985) Langzeitergebnisse der transluminalen koronaren Angioplastie von chronischen Herzkranzgefäßverschlüssen. Z Kardiol 74: 309
22. Meier B, King SB, Grüntzig AR, Douglas JS, Hollman J, Ischinger T, Galan K, Tankersley R (1984) Repeat coronary angioplasty. J Am Coll Cardiol 4: 463
23. Meier B (1984) Kissing balloon coronary angioplasty. Am J Cardiol 54: 918
24. Meyer J, Merx W, Schmitz H, Erbel R., Kiesslich T, Dörr R, Lambertz H, Bethge C, Krebs W, Bardos P, Minale C, Messmer BJ, Effert S (1982) Percutaneous transluminal coronary angioplasty immediately after intracoronary streptolysis of transmural myocardial infarction. Circulation 66: 905
25. Meyer J, Schmitz H, Kiesslich T, Erbel R, Krebs W, Schulz W, Bardos P, Minale C, Messmer BJ, Effert S (1983) Percutaneous transluminal coronary angioplasty in patients with stable and unstable angina pectoris: analysis of early and late results. Am Heart J 106: 973
26. Mizuno K, Kurita A, Imazeki N (1984) Pathological findings after percutaneous transluminal coronary angioplasty. Br Heart J 52: 588
27. Mock MB, Holmes DR, Vlietstra RE, Gersh BJ, Detre KM, Kelsey SF, Orszulak TA, Schaff HV, Piehler JM, van Raden MJ, Passamani ER, Kent KM, Grüntzig AR (1984) Percutaneous transluminal coronary angioplasty (PTCA) in the elderly patient: experience in the National Heart, Lung and Blood Institute PTC registry Am J Cardiol 53 [Suppl]: 89C
28. National Heart, Lung and Blood Institute (1983) Proceedings of the Workshop on the outcome of percutaneous transluminal coronary angioplasty. Am J Cardiol 53 [Suppl]: 1C-146C (1984)
29 Raizner AE, Hust RG, Lewis JM, Winters WL, Batty JW, Roberts R (1986) Transluminal coronary angioplasty in the elderly. Am J Cardiol 57: 29
30. Schmutzler H, Rutsch W (1983) Die transluminale Koronar-Dilatation. Internist 24: 402
31. Serruys PW, Umans V, Heyndrickx GR, v.d. Brand M, de Feyter PJ, Wijns W, Jaski B, Hugenholtz PG (1985) Elective PTCA of totally occluded coronary arteries not associated with acute myocardial infarction; short-term and long-term results. Eur Heart J 5: 2
32. Simpson JB, Robert N, Baim D, Harrison DC (1981) Clinical experience with a new catheter system for percutaneous transluminal coronary angioplasty. Am J Cardiol 47: 395
33. Simpson JB, Baim DS, Robert EW, Harrison DC (1982) A new catheter system for coronary angioplasty. Am J Cardiol 49: 1216
34. Stertzer SH, Myler RK, Insel H, Wallsh E, Rossi P (1985) Percutaneous transluminal coronary angioplasty in left main stem coronary stenosis: a five-year appraisal. Int J Cardiol 9: 149
35. Waller BF, McManus BM, Gorfinkel H, Kishel JC, Schmidt EC, Kent KM, Roberts WC (1983) Status of the major epicardial coronary arteries 80 to 150 days after percutaneous transluminal coronary angioplasty Am J Cardiol 52: 81
36. Wood WG (1982) Transluminal coronary angioplasty. N Engl J Med 306: 1055

Authors'address:
Dr. B. Höfling
Medizinische Klinik I
Klinikum Großhadern
Marchioninistr. 15
8000 München 70
West Germany

Early and Late Results After Percutaneous Transluminal Coronary Angioplasty Compared with Bypass Operation

G. Kober, C. Vallbracht, and M. Kaltenbach

Center for Internal Medicine, Dept. of Cardiology, Univ. Hospital,
Frankfurt a. M., Federal Republic of Germany

Transluminal coronary angioplasty (PTCA) as a procedure for improving coronary circulation was adopted into the therapy of coronary heart disease in 1977, 9 years after the description of aortocoronary bypass graft surgery by Favoloro [7]. Although it has been in use for a shorter period of time, angioplasty is already a real alternative to coronary bypass graft surgery for an increasing number of patients.

A true comparison between the results of these very different procedures is hardly possible, for several reasons. Aortocoronary bypass graft surgery is now technically fully developed, nearly 20 years after its introduction into therapy, while PTCA is still experiencing rapid technical improvements, its use is spreading quickly, and experience is increasing significantly. A comparison of two methods that are in different states of development does not seem rational. However, a comparison of the results of the first 9 years of coronary bypass graft therapy and those of angioplasty would not provide any information on the *present* effectiveness of both procedures.

The patients who have been treated with the two procedures to date are hardly comparable, as angioplasty is used for about 70% of patients with single-vessel disease. Today, single-vessel disease is rarely an indication of aortocoronary bypass graft surgery, which is primarily performed in patients with multiple-vessel disease. But even with multiple-vessel disease, an increasing tendency to perform balloon dilatation can be recognized.

Results of Coronary Angioplasty

In Frankfurt, 1453 angioplasty procedures were performed between October 1977 and October 1985. Of the first 1000 operations 73% were in patients with single-vessel disease and 27% in patients with double- or triple-vessel disease. The majority of interventions were performed on the left anterior descending coronary artery. Thirty-six percent of the patients had already suffered myocardial infarction, but in most cases it was not transmural (Table 1).

The success rate increased from 58% for the first 100 operations to 84% for operations 701 to 1000. Emergency coronary bypass graft surgery had to be performed in 5.2% of the patients. Following the introduction of the long-wire steerable technique there seems to be a reduction in the complication rate, with 4.2% of patients having undergone emergency bypass graft surgery among 540 recent procedures. The mortality for the first 1000 operations was 0.30% (Table 2).

Table 1. Findings in 1000 patients before PTCA

Finding	%
Single-vessel disease (SVD)	73
Double-vessel disease (DVD)	18
Triple-vessel disease (TVD)	9
LAD	69
Right coronary artery	19
Left circumflex	8
Left main	1
Bypass graft	3
State after myocardial infarction	36
Transmural infarction	23
Nontransmural infarction	77
Infarction in SVD	34
Infarction in DVD	46
Infarction in TVD	40
Angioplasty of infarct-related vessel	85

Table 2. Results of 1000 coronary angioplasty procedures

Result	%
Success rate for:	
1000 procedures	77
Procedures 1- 100	58
Procedures 101- 700	76
Procedures 701-1000	84
Emergency bypass surgery	5.2
Mortality	0.3

Follow-up investigations including ergometry and angiograms were routinely performed in all patients, 3 and 12 months after the procedure. Of 439 follow-up angiograms, 17.4% showed restenoses. The patients who had their first procedure in a native vessel showed a restenosis rate of 15%; the majority of restenosis developed within the first 3 months. Higher recurrence rates were observed in patients with repeat angioplasty procedures (33%), dilatation of bypass stenoses (45%), and angioplasty of chronic coronary artery occlusions (54%). The preceding data, especially the restenosis rates, were obtained exclusively from angiographic follow-up investigations [3, 4]. The clinical and exercise electrocardiographic findings are more favorable. Thus, a great number of patients who developed a restenosis were symptomatically improved. Frequently, the degree of recurrent stenosis was below the predilatation degree.

Angiographic long-term results in 22 patients are shown in Fig. 1. In all 22 patients a third angiographic study was performed at a mean of 42 months after angioplasty. The

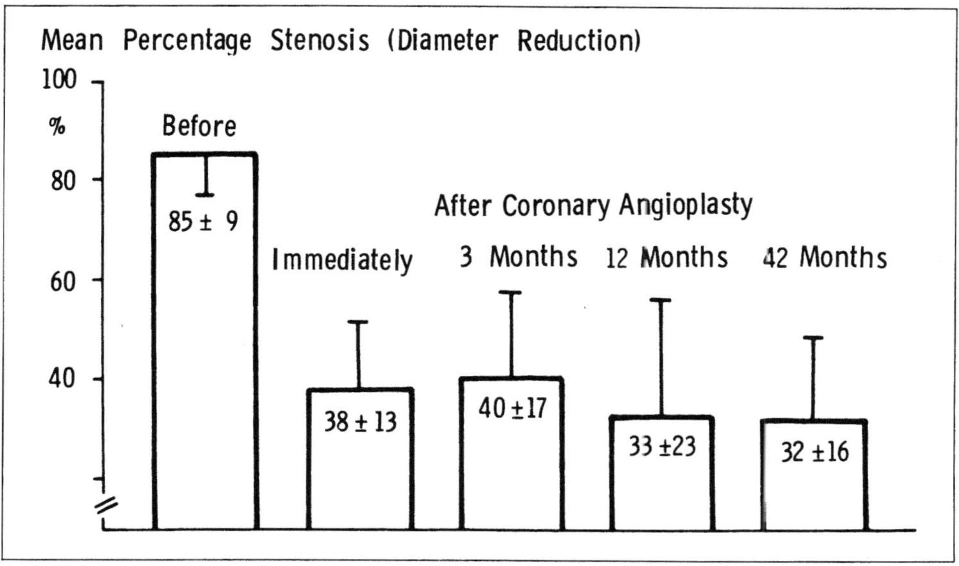

Fig. 1. Long-term results of coronary angioplasty in 22 patients

mean percentage stenosis was reduced from 85% to 38% by PTCA. Three months later it was 40% and at 12 months, 33%.

None of the patients developed an increase in the remaining stenosis by more than 10% within the following 2-6 years. The mean percentage stenosis remained unchanged at 32%. Due to progression of the underlying disease, new stenoses in other vessels or vessel segments developed in five patients; these were treated again successfully by PTCA in four. .

According to the literature on the angiographically assessed patency rate of bypass grafts, the frequency of early occlusions (within 4-12 weeks) is about 10%, that of occlusions within the 1st year after the operation about 20%. In the following years a further occlusion rate of only 2% is reported.

Thus, the bypass occlusion rate is close to the rate of restenosis after PTCA. But, again, the limited significance of such a historical comparison has to be mentioned. At present, no studies are available on comparable patient groups treated in a random manner with either of the procedures. Nor is it likely that such investigations will be performed in the future, as the long-term success of angioplasty is proven.

We do not yet have the results of a study being conducted in our clinic to compare complications and long-term success of angioplasty treatment in our patient population with single bypass operations performed mainly in other clinics. However, a comparison between two not completely identical patient populations from a study performed at Emory University in Atlanta, USA, in 1984 [2] showed a mortality of 0.8% for the aortocoronary bypass graft surgery and no mortality at all for the angioplasty-treated group. Newly developed Q waves appeared in 2.7% of the patients after angioplasty (including 20 patients who underwent emergency bypass graft surgery) and in 3.6% of those selected for bypass grafts, thus implying a fairly similar infarction rate secondary to both methods.

Comparable data are available for nonidentical patient groups after angioplasty and coronary bypass surgery in terms of complete vocational rehabilitation and duration of the patients' sick leave after the operation. In our own patient population, comprising 54 patients with angioplasty and 52 with aortocoronary bypass graft surgery, the percentage of patients who returned to work after angioplasty was markedly higher (61%) than that following aortocoronary bypass graft surgery (25%) [6]. In contrast, Meier et al. in Geneva [5] and Boulay et al. in Montreal [1] did not find any differences, the rate of patients returning to work being, on the whole, markedly higher than that in our patient population.

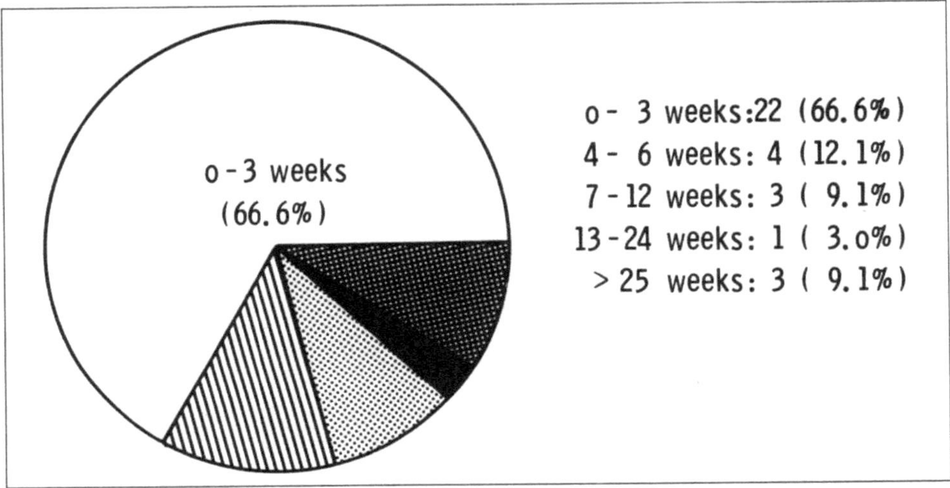

Fig. 2a. Period of occupational disability following PTCA

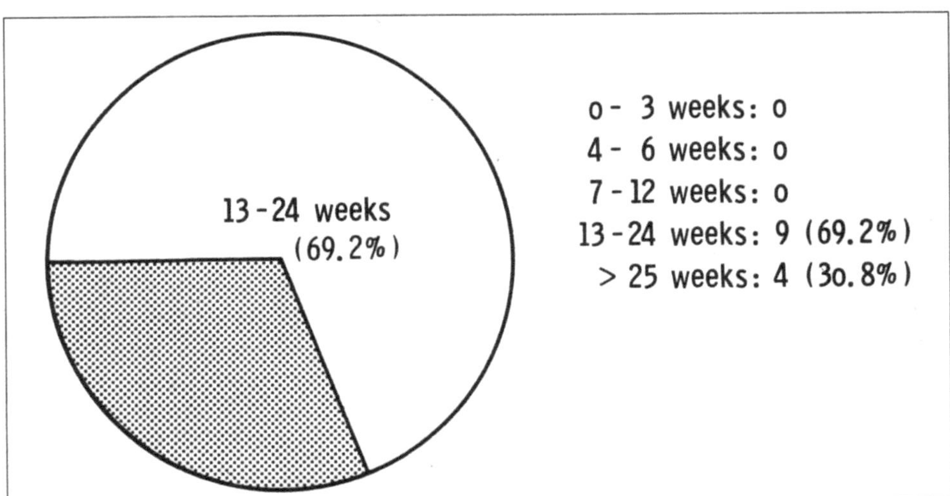

Fig. 2b. Period of occupational disability following bypass surgery

It is doubtful whether these differences can be explained by differently composed patient populations. They may be attributable to health insurance systems or different attitudes of patients and physicians toward the disease, and even job-market factors may play a role.

There is no question about the fact that the amount of time the patient is on sick leave differs considerably for the two methods. In the mean, our patients returned to work 7.4 weeks following angioplasty, whereas it took a mean of 38.1 weeks, i.e., five times longer, until patients returned to work following a bypass operation. After angioplasty 66.6% of the patients returned to work within 3 weeks (Fig. 2a), while 69.2% of the patients who had undergone bypass surgery returned to work between weeks 13 and 24, the remaining patients much later (Fig. 2b).

Conclusions

Angioplasty and aortocoronary bypass graft surgery are not competitive procedures. PTCA is the therapy of choice for patients with one stenosis that requires revascularization. Coronary bypass graft surgery is performed predominantly in patients with multiple-vessel disease. However, in this patient group the applicability of the two types of therapy may overlap.

If one tries to compare both procedures one should be aware of the differences between the patient populations and of the different periods of experience with these two methods. In different patient groups the immediate and short-term success rates, i.e., the patency rate of dilated arteries and bypass grafts, and the perioperative infarction rates and mortalities are comparable. The numbers of patients who are clinically improved and whose exercise ECG shows improved exercise tolerance do not differ.

Long-term results over 5 years or more in a larger group of patients are not available to date, due to the still limited experience with PTCA. The long-term success rate is greatly influenced by the progression of the underlying disease. Our long-term experience with angioplasty is restricted to a limited number of angiographic restudies which have shown no local restenosis later than 12 months after successful angioplasty. Should a study of a greater number of patients confirm this preliminary result, this would imply that on this point at least, angioplasty has an advantage over aortocoronary bypass graft surgery.

While it is doubtful whether the percentages of patients who return to work after both procedures differ, it is clear that the length of hospitalization and disease-induced sick leave is markedly longer after aortocoronary bypass graft surgery – in our patient population by a factor of 5.

Further facts that are clearly in favor of angioplasty, such as the economic and psychological aspects, do not fall within the scope of this report.

References

1. Boulay F, David P, David PR, Bourassa MG (1985) Work status and percutaneous transluminal coronary angioplasty. In: Walter PJ (ed) Return to work after coronary artery bypass surgery. Springer-Verlag, Berlin Heidelberg New York Tokyo, pp 183-190

2. Jones EL, Murphy DA, Craver JM 1984) Comparison of coronary artery bypass surgery and percutaneous transluminal coronary angioplasty including surgery for failed angioplasty. Am Heart J 107: 830-835
3. Kaltenbach M, Kober G, Scherer D, Vallbracht C (1985) Recurrence rate after successful coronary angioplasty. Eur Heart J 6: 276-281
4. Kober G, Hopf R, Reinemer H, Kaltenbach M (1985) Langzeitergebnisse der transluminalen koronaren Angioplastie von chronischen Herzkranzgefäßverschlüssen. Z Kardiol 74: 309-316
5. Meier B, Chaves V, v. Segesser L, Faidutti B, Rutishauser W (1985) Vocational rehabilitation after coronary angioplasty and coronary bypass surgery. In: Walter PJ (ed) Return to work after coronary artery bypass surgery. Springer-Verlag, Berlin Heidelberg New York Toyko, pp 171–176
6. Vallbracht C, Kober G, Scherer D, Kaltenbach M (1985) Return to work after coronary angioplasty. In: Walter PJ (ed) Return to work after coronary artery bypass surgery. Springer-Verlag, Berlin Heidelberg New York Tokyo, pp 177-182
7. Favoloro R G (1968) Saphenous vein autograft replacement of severe segmental artery occlusion. Ann Thorac Surg 5: 334

Author's address:
Prof. Dr. med. G. Kober
Abteilung für Kardiologie
Zentrum der Inneren Medizin
Universitätsklinikum
Theodor-Stern-Kai 7
D-6000 Frankfurt a. M. 70
West Germany

Detection of Ischemia during PTCA with Extended Electrocardiographic Monitoring

T. von Arnim, A. Stäblein, and B. Höfling

Medizinische Klinik I, Klinikum Großhadern der Ludwig-Maximilians-Universität München, Federal Republic of Germany

Introduction

Monitoring of signs of ischemia during PTCA is important for judging both the acute and the cumulative effects of repeated coronary occlusions on the myocardium. In animals, repeated brief periods of ischemia have been shown to cause cumulative damage which may lead to myocardial necrosis [2]. Ischemic changes during coronary angioplasty in man have mostly been monitored with single limb-leads. More sophisticated studies have utilized pulmonary wedge pressure monitoring [6], echocardiographic imaging [4, 5], or electrocardiographic recordings from the guide wire [8] to detect and follow transient ischemic changes. The most practicable and well-known technique for detecting myocardial ischemia, i.e., the normal ECG with chest leads, has not been tried because of the obstruction imposed by metal leads on the fluoroscopic view. In our laboratory we developed chest leads for the ECG which are made from very thin, wound wires and do not disturb the fluoroscopic image. They nevertheless allow a full chest lead recording throughout the procedure. The present study was undertaken to assess the sensitivity of chest lead ECG monitoring during coronary angioplasty and to compare it with limb-lead monitoring and with the pain perceived by the patient.

Methods

Patient characteristics are described in Table 1. In 50 patients a total of 217 dilatations were performed. In 172 of these dilatations and clear temporal coordination of balloon inflation, balloon deflation, and the corresponding ECG was possible. These 172 dilatations, i.e., the recordings of limb leads, chest leads, and patients' chest pain, have been evaluated for this study.
Dilatation time was 39.1 ± 15.4 s (mean $\pm$ SD) and dilatation pressure was 7 ± 2.0 atm. The dilatation technique was as described by Grüntzig [7], and we utilized Schneider-Grüntzig and ACS catheter material and wires.
Our chest lead electrodes were made from thin, wound aluminum wires. The wires used for this study represent a further development from an electrode system described earlier for the same purpose [1]. Figure 1 shows three different electrodes with wires and a balloon catheter for comparison. Figure 2a shows the same electrodes under fluoroscopy, and it can be seen that wire no. 3 is completely translucent. Figure 2b shows a fluorosco-

pic view during the PTCA procedure with chest leads – model no. 3 – mounted. Only the buttons of the self-adhesive electrodes are seen.

An example of a full chest-lead recording during coronary balloon dilatation is shown in Fig. 3. A few seconds after the beginning of balloon inflation the first ST-T changes can be observed; these increase in severity and in the number of leads involved and then decrease gradually after balloon deflation.

Table 1. Characteristics of the 50 consecutive patients studied

Age (mean ± SD)	52.2 ± 9.5 years	
Sex distribution	male 36 (72%) female 14 (28%)	
previous myocardial infarction:		
no M1		24 (48%)
anterior M1		24 (48%)
posterior M1		2 (4%)
coronary vessel dilated:		
proximal left anterior descendent (LAD)		23 (46%)
mid/distal left anterior descendent (LAD 2/3)		18 (36%)
left circumflex (LCX)		7 (14%)
right coronary artery (RCA)		2 (4%)
severity of coronary stenoses:		
I (≤ 75%)		4 (8%)
II (≤ 90%)		13 (26%)
III (≤ 99%)		22 (44%)
IV (≤ 100%)		11 (22%)

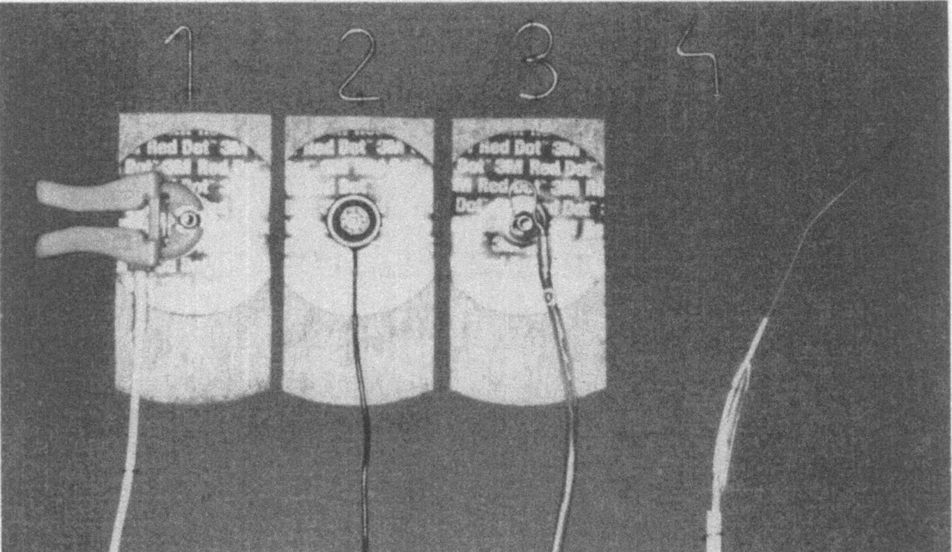

Fig. 1. Three different types of electrocardiographic electrodes used for monitoring purposes, with a balloon catheter for comparison. Wire no. 3 is our radiolucent lead

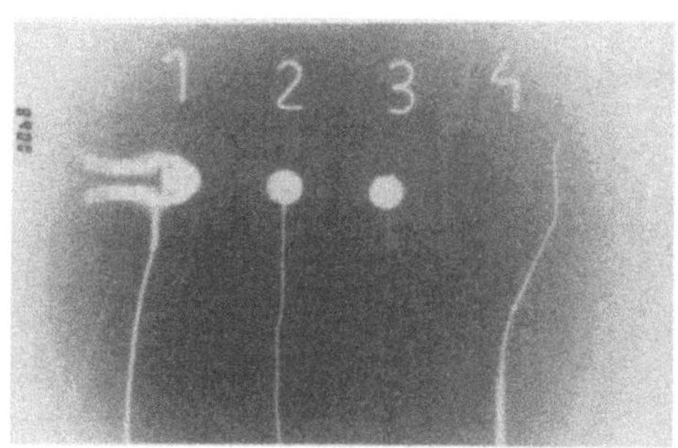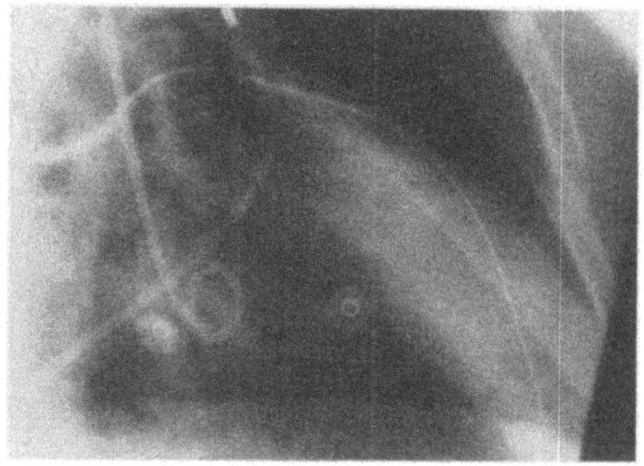

Fig. 2a. The same electrodes and wires as in Fig. 1. Wire no. 3 is completely radiolucent. **b** Fluoroscopic image during the PTCA procedure with our chest lead system mounted. Only the buttons of the electrodes can be seen, and they do not disturb the fluoroscopic view

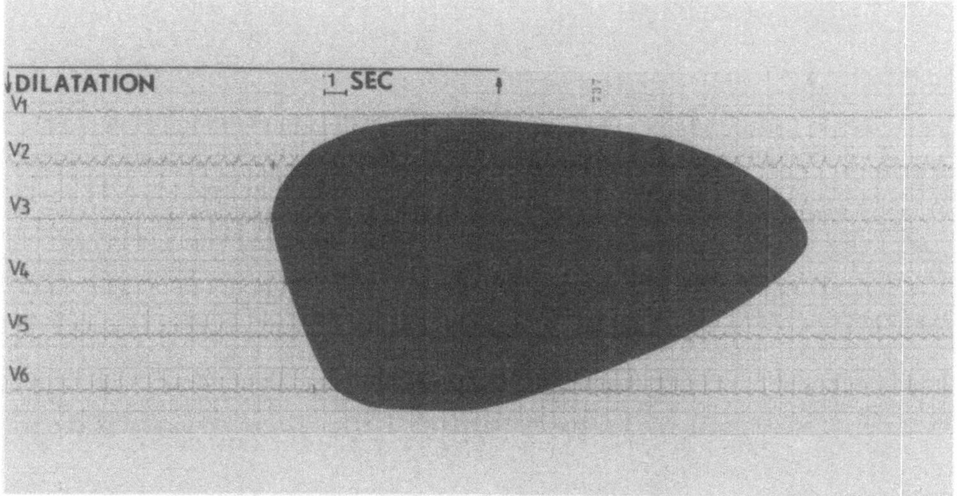

Fig. 3. Full chest-lead recording with ischemic changes during intracoronary balloon dilatation. There is a temporal and local spread of ST-T changes at the beginning and end of ischemia.

For each dilatation the following data were collected: (a) time and pressure of balloon inflation; (b) time from balloon inflation to first ECG changes, duration of ECG changes, time from balloon deflation to disappearance of ECG changes; (c) time from balloon inflation to appearance of chest pain; (d) grading of maximal observed ECG changes following a simple grading scheme (Fig. 4). All ECG evaluations were done in comparison with changes observed with the chest leads V1-V6 and limb leads I-III.

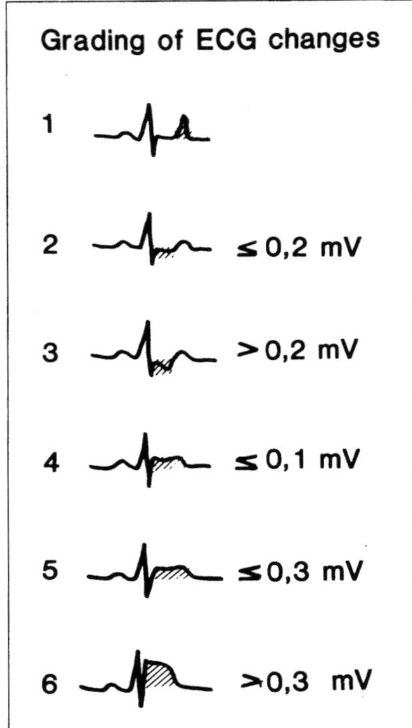

Fig. 4. For comparison ST- and T-wave changes as observed on the chest lead and limb lead ECGs were grouped in a rough grading scheme with increasing severity of changes. Synchronous changes in chest and limb leads could be analyzed during single dilatations.

Results

Of 172 dilatations, 79 (46%) were performed in the proximal LAD, 62 (36%) in the mid and distal portions of the LAD, 24 (14%) in the LCX and seven (4%) in the RCA. A primary success as judged by standard criteria [7] was achieved in 85% of the 50 patients treated.

During 53 of 172 dilatations (31%) no electrocardiographic changes were observed in either lead system. In 91 of 172 dilatations (53%) transient ST-T changes were observed in both the chest leads V1-V6 and the limb leads I-III. In 28 of 172 dilatations (16%), however, there were transient ST-T changes only in the chest leads V1-V6. Thus, with chest lead monitoring during the PTCA procedure approximately one third more ECG changes can be observed than with limb-lead monitoring alone.

Figure 5 is a correlation graph for comparison of the time lag between balloon inflation and first appearance of ischemic ECG changes in the two lead systems tested. The points in the graph represent the 91 dilatations which caused ECG changes in both V1-V6 and I-III. The diagonal line is the line of symmetry, i.e., each point on the line means that changes appeared on both lead systems at the same time. There is a considerable degree of scatter around this line, but the means for appearance times are not far apart: 15 ± 7 s for leads V1-V6 and 17 ± 7 s for leads I-III (difference not significant).

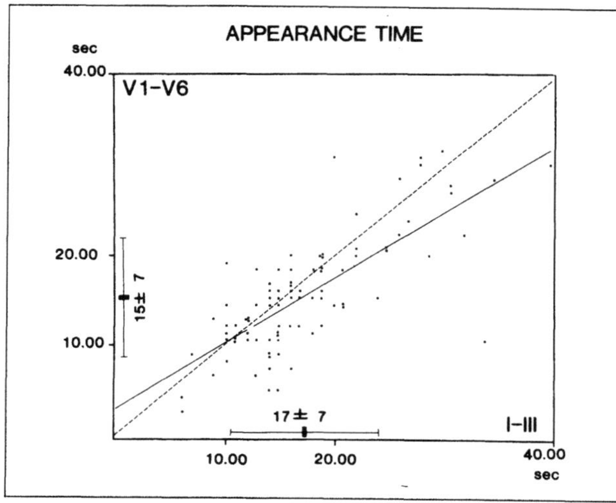

Fig. 5. Time for appearance of ischemic ST-T changes after balloon inflation. *y-axis:* Chest leads V1-V6; *x-axis:* limb leads I-III. The mean appearance times are 15-17 s and not significantly different for the two lead systems

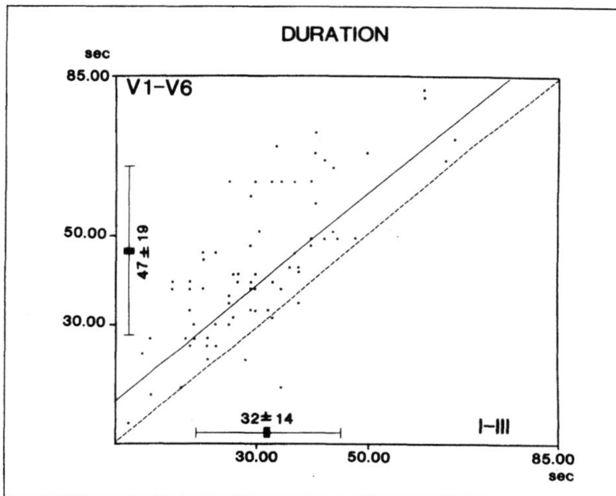

Fig. 6. Duration of ischemic ST-T changes. The duration is considerably longer with chest leads for all dilatations which would be compared. Thus chest-lead monitoring affords increased sensitivity for prolonged or cumulative ischemia

The duration of ischemic ECG changes in both lead systems are compared in Figure 6. There is a clear shift of the regression line for the correlation upward from the line of symmetry. This means longer detectability of ischemic changes with chest leads, and the parallel shift shows that it is equally pronounced for shorter and longer periods of ischemia. The equation for the regression is:

$$y = 13.16 + 0.99x$$

The mean duration of ischemic changes in the chest leads is 47 ± 19 s vs 32 ± 14 s for the limb leads. This difference is significant ($\underline{P} < 0.001$). When the severity of ischemic

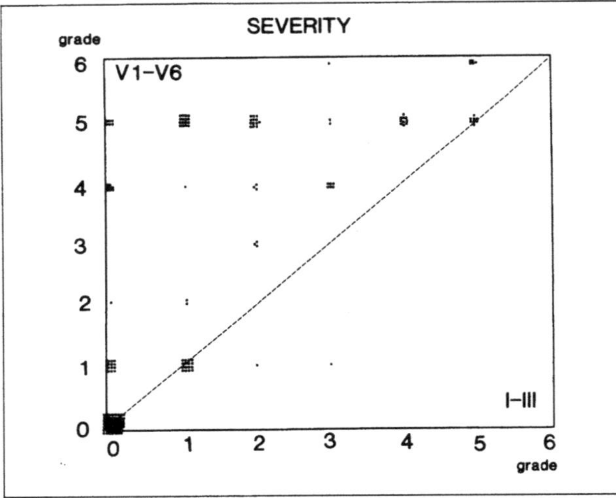

Fig. 7. Comparison of severity of ischemic ST-T changes in both lead systems. Most points lie to the left of the line of symmetry; i.e., chest leads show more severe changes, mostly ST elevations

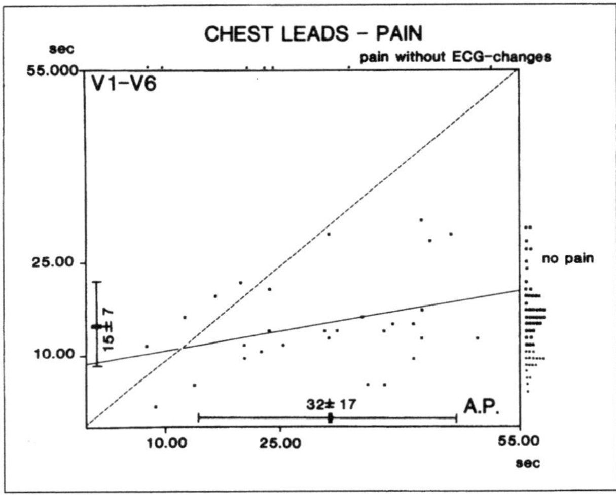

Fig. 8. Comparison of appearance time of ST-T changes in chest leads and onset of angina. Pain comes considerably later, and in a great number of dilatations there is no pain at all (59/172) despite evidence of ischemia from the ECG

ECG changes is grouped according to the scheme of Fig. 4 in both lead systems and plotted together, the scatter graph of Fig. 7 is obtained. It is obvious that most points lie in the upper left part of the graph; this is due to higher grades of severity – especially ST elevation – in chest leads, where limb leads show only T-wave changes or ST depression. This asymmetry is also highly significant ($\underline{P} < 0.001$).

Besides the ECG changes, which were continuously recorded, we recorded the onset of pain in the chest after balloon inflation in all patients. They were asked repeatedly to state to the catheter team when angina started, became more severe, or subsided. Figure 8 shows the correlation of time of onset of ECG changes in leads V1-V6 vs. time of onset of

32

pain. With a large scatter, pain comes much later than ECG changes, 32 ± 17 s vs. 15 ± 7 s ($\underline{P} < 0.001$). In a large number of dilatations (59/172) no pain was perceived by the patient despite electrocardiographic evidence of ischemia.

Discussion

During PTCA the most careful monitoring of ischemia is mandatory to detect early and with certainty any prolonged or unexpected appearances of ischemia. During occlusion of the vessel the appearance of signs of ischemia is an expected event, and its precocity and severity are representative of the size of the area at risk and its collateral perfusion. Yet after deflation of the balloon the disappearance of signs of ischemia and pain is even more important, because it reassures the operator of the re-establishment of antegrade flow through the vessel that is being dilated. For instance, if ischemic ECG changes persist after balloon deflation, this could be the first sign of an acute occlusion. Also, prolonged recovery time of the transiently ischemic myocardium after dilatation can be detected by sensitive monitoring.

Most centers are used to the monitoring of limb leads during cardiac catheterization, and this type of procedure is also followed during PTCA [7]. However, more sensitive or more meaningful methods are under investigation for this purpose: continuous recording of coronary potassium concentration [11], recording of ventricular filling with a nuclear probe [9], two-dimensional echocardiography [4, 5], or recording of pulmonary capillary wedge pressure [6].

We have developed a method that seems practical, as the problem of obstruction of the visual field by ECG leads has been solved. The specificity – i.e., that transient ST-T changes during transient coronary occlusion are of ischemic origin – is not questionable. Thus, we have investigated the sensitivity of our lead system as compared with that of the limb leads. We found a considerably higher sensitivity for the chest leads, as there are approximately one third more dilatations which show ECG changes when chest leads are recorded. The appearance times were not very different for the two methods, and other investigators have also found the first evidence of ischemia 15-20 s after balloon inflation [4, 5]. The chest leads showed evidence of ischemia for about 15 s longer than limb leads. This can be important, because it may be unwise to re-occlude a vessel when the myocardium that is dependent on this vessel has not yet recovered from the preceding balloon occlusion. Thus, improved detection of ischemia may make repeated dilatations safer.

The occurrence of cardiac pain during angioplasty was a much later and less sensitive marker of ischemia. A considerable number of dilatations were performed without pain but did show clear ECG changes. These painless but obviously ischemic episodes are classic examples of "silent ischemia", which is recognized increasingly also in other circumstances in coronary patients [3].

Nevertheless, pain remains an impressive if fallible marker of ischemia, especially when it subsides promptly after balloon deflation, but if taken as the only sign of ischemia it would be too un-reliable. In conclusion, our study shows that chest lead monitoring during PTCA is feasible and provides sensitive markers of ischemia. Compared with other methods of more intensive monitoring for ischemia the continuous recording of a chest lead ECG has the advantages of much less operator and technical expense combined with a highly sensitive signal that is familiar to any cardiologist.

References

1. von Arnim T, Kemkes B, Höfling B (1985) Monitoring of myocardial ischaemia during PTCA. Improved sensitivity with 12-lead ECG. In: Meyer J, Erbel R, Rupprecht HJ (eds) Improvement of myocardial perfusion. Thrombolysis, angioplasty, bypass surgery. Martinus Nijhoff Publishers, The Hague, pp 186–189
2. Geft JL, Fishbein MC, Ninomiya K (1982) Intermittent brief periods of ischemia have a cumulative effect and may cause myocardial necrosis. Circulation 66: 1150–1153
3. Gottlieb SO, Ouyang P, Mellits ED, Gerstenblith G (1985) Silent ischemia during medical therapy predicts unfavorable outcomes in unstable angina. Circulation [Suppl III] 649: 163
4. Hauser AM, Ramos RG, Gordon S, Timmis GC, Dudlets P (1985) Sequence of mechanical electrocardiographic and clinical effects of repeated coronary artery occlusion in human beings: echocardiographic observations during coronary angioplasty. J Am Coll Cardiol 5 (2): 193-197
5. Henkel B, Erbel R, Clas W, Schreiner C, Kopp H, Pop T, Meyer J (1985) Acute changes of myocardial function by PTCA. Evaluation by two-dimensional echocardiography. In: Meyer J, Erbel R, Rupprecht HJ (eds) Improvement of myocardial perfusion. Martinus Nijhoff, The Hague, pp
6. Herrmann G, Simon R, Amende I, Lichtlen PR (1985) EKG und pulmonaler Kapillardruck als Ischämieparameter während Ballondilatation. Z Kardiol [Suppl III] 171: 51
7. King S, Douglas JS, Grüntzig AR (1985) Percutaneous transluminal coronary angioplasty. In: King SB, Douglas JS (eds) Coronary arteriography and angioplasty. McGraw-Hill, New York, pp 433-460
8. Meier P, Kilisch JP, Adette JJ, Casalini P, Rutishauser W (1985) Intracoronary electrocardiogram, coronary wedge pressure and collaterals during angioplasty. Circulation [Suppl III] 875: 219
9. Monteferrante JC, Stein JH, Ro JH, Blake JW, McCrossan J, Bontemps RA, Herman MV, Weiss MB (1984) Systolic and diastolic left ventricular function by nuclear probe during transluminal coronary angioplasty. Circulation [Suppl III] 146: 37
10. Sherman CT, Litvack F, Grundfest W, Lee MF, Kass R, Swan HJC, Matloff J, Forrester JS (1985) Fiberoptic coronary angioscopy identifies thrombus in all patients with unstable angina. Circulation [Suppl III] 446: 112
11. Webb SC, Rickards AF, Poole-Wilson PA (1983) Coronary sinus potassium concentration recorded during coronary angioplasty. Br Heart I 50: 146-148

Authors' address:
Priv.-Doz. Dr. T. von Arnim
Klinikum Großhadern
Medizinische Klinik I
Marchioninistraße 15
8000 München 70

Effect of Coronary Occlusion During Percutaneous Transluminal Angioplasty on Systolic and Diastolic Left Ventricular Function, Coronary Hemodynamics, and Myocardial Energetic Metabolism

P. W. Serruys, F. Piscione[1], W. Wijns[2], J. A. J. Hegge, E. Harmsen[3],
M. van den Brand, P. de Feyter, J. W. de Jong, P. G. Hugenholtz
Catheterization and Cardiochemical Laboratories, Thoraxcenter,
Erasmus University, Rotterdam, The Netherlands

Introduction

Until recently, the measurement in man of left ventricular geometry and hemodynamics and the assessment of alteration in myocardial metabolism early after an abrupt occlusion of a major coronary artery were not feasible. Percutaneous transluminal coronary angioplasty (PTCA), however, now provides a unique opportunity to study the time course of these variables during the transient interruption of coronary flow in the balloon occlusion sequence in patients with single-vessel disease and without angiographically demonstrable collateral circulation [1, 2].

The need to detect any persisting metabolic or mechanical dysfunction becomes of even greater concern as the number of dilated vessels and the duration of balloon inflation tend to increase, thereby increasing both the extent and the severity of ischemia. The risk exists that the damage induced by the intervention may exceed its benefit. We report here the dynamic changes in left ventricular hemodynamics and the concurrent left ventricular geometry changes assessed by angiography in 14 patients during PTCA. This study was undertaken in order to investigate the sequence of events during transient ischemia induced by transluminal angioplasty and to determine whether the effects of ischemia after repeated occlusions were reversible or not.

In another group of 28 patients, blood flow, lactate, and hypoxanthine metabolism were analyzed during reactive hyperemia after repeated occlusions of the left anterior descending coronary artery; the effects of ischemia proved quickly reversible but were indicative of impending cellular dysfunction.

---

[1] Dr. Piscione is supported by CNR-NATO research fellowship no. 216.1095; present address: Clinica Medica I, II Policlinico, Via S. Pansini, 80131, Napoli, Italy

[2] Present address: Laboratory of Nuclear Medicine, UCLA School of Medicine, Los Angeles, CA 90024, U.S.A.

[3] Present address: Department of Biochemistry, South Parkroad, Oxford OX1 3QV, United Kingdom

Study Population and Protocol (Study I)

Fourteen patients were selected from 356 consecutive attempted angioplasty procedures. These patients met the criteria of an isolated obstructive lesion of one coronary vessel (left anterior descending artery in ten patients, right coronary in four, left circumflex in one) having a normal resting left ventricular function and wall motion. Four patients had mild essential hypertension and elevated left ventricular filling pressures (EDP 25 mmHg). During the PTCA procedure the number of transluminal occlusions performed per patient was 4.9 ± 2.2 (mean ± SD).

The average duration of each occlusion was 51 ± 12 s (mean ± SD), and the total occlusion time during the whole procedure was 252 ± 140 s (mean ± SD). Pressures were recorded with a tip manometer 8-F pigtail catheter, and derived variables were calculated off-line by a computer system [3, 4].

Three to four ventriculograms (30 degrees RAO at 50 frames/s) were obtained by injection of 0.75 ml/kg of a nonionic contrast medium (metrizamide, Amipaque). The hemodynamic and angiographic investigations were performed before the PTCA procedure was begun, after 20 s of occlusion during the second dilatation, after 50 s of occlusion during the fourth dilatation, and again 5 min after completion of the PTCA procedure. These sequential LV angiograms were made only after the values for left ventricular end-diastolic pressure and the various isovolumic parameters had returned to the levels these recorded before the initial angiogram. In all cases, the interval between any two angiograms was at least 10 min. Care was taken to maintain the patient's position unchanged in relation to the X-ray equipment during the consecutive angiograms. Diaphragm movement was reduced to a minimum by instructing the patient to inspire shallowly with care to prevent the Valsalva maneuver.

Analysis of Pressure-derived Indices During Systole and Diastole

Left ventricular pressure was measured with a Millar micromanometer catheter and digitized at 250 samples/s. Combined analog and digital filtering resulted in an effective time constant of less than 10 ms. This employed an updated version of the beat-to-beat program described previously [3, 4].

Peak LV pressure, LV end-diastolic pressure, peak negative dP/dt, peak positive dP/dt, and the relation between dP/dt/P and P linearly extrapolated to $P = 0$ (V_{max}) were computed on-line after a data acquisition of 20 s.

Determination of Relaxation Parameters

A new technique has been implemented for the off-line beat-to-beat calculation of the relaxation parameters [5, 6, 7], using a semilogarithmic model:

$P(t) = P_0 e^{-t/T}$. The Po and T parameters are estimated from a linear least-squares fit of $LnP = -t/T + LnP_0$, starting from the time of peak $-dP/dt$.

a) fit of first 40 ms   ($n = 8$), T1, bi-exponential [7],
b) fit after the first 40 ms ($n = 8$), T2, bi-exponential [7],
c) fit of all points   ($n = 8$), T, mono-exponential.

A complete cardiac cycle was analyzed frame by frame from all cineangiograms. The ventricular contour was detected automatically [8]. For each analyzed cineframe left ventricular volume was computed according to Simpson's rule. After the end-diastolic and end-systolic frames were determined, stroke volume, global ejection fraction and total cardiac index were computed. End-diastolic (ED) pressure was defined as that point on the pressure trace at which the derivative of the pressure first exceeded 200 mmHg/s [3], and in all cases it coincided with the maximal measured LV volume. End-systole (ES) was defined, with reference to the pressure tracing, as the occurrence of the dicrotic notch of the central aortic pressure.

Study Population and Protocol (Study II)

Twenty-eight patients were studied: 21 men and seven women, aged from 38 to 74 years. Of these, 16 were in NYHA class II, eight in class III, and four in class IV. In all the ejection fraction was greater than 50%. These 28 patients were selected from 58 patients in whom thermodilution coronary sinus blood flow was measured during angioplasty for various indications. They were chosen because they required at least four transluminal dilatations. These four dilations were performed with a total duration of occlusion of 192 ± 40 s (mean ± SD).
All patients in this study gave their informed consent, and there were no complications directly related to the research procedure.

PTCA Technique

Percutaneous transluminal coronary angioplasty was performed by the same technique in all patients. Via a 9-F, 16-cm introducing sheath, a guiding catheter was directed into the stenotic area under fluoroscopic and pressure control. PTCA was performed according to the technique of Grüntzig, with the equipment of Schneider, via the femoral route. In all cases the pressure gradient across the obstructive lesion was recorded before, during, and after balloon inflation. The dilatation catheters were either the 20–30 or 20–37 models. The inflation pressure ranged from 2 to 12 atm, while individual dilatations ranged from 40 to 60 s. Attempts to dilate the lesion were repeated as long as the gradient persisted. Coronary angiography with nonionic contrast medium (metrizamide) was performed immediately before and after PTCA. Lateral, anteroposterior, oblique, and hemiaxial angiographic views were obtained in all patients.

Flow Measurements

A thermodilution coronary sinus blood flow catheter (Webster) was introduced into the coronary sinus by way of a right brachial vein. In 15 cases the catheter tip was placed in the great cardiac vein. Coronary sinus blood flow (13 patients, group I) or great cardiac vein blood flow (15 patients, group II) was measured by the continuous thermodilution method before and after the PTCA procedure, as well as during each transluminal occlusion. At the beginning of the investigation the location of the external thermistor, in the coronary sinus or in the great cardiac vein, was verified by injection of 3 ml of contrast medium. Each recording of blood flow during coronary angioplasty began before balloon inflation and was interrupted at the moment of balloon deflation.

Coronary vascular resistance (CVR) was calculated for great cardiac vein (GCV) or coronary sinus (CS) [9] using the mean arterial pressure (MAP) and blood flow in the great cardiac vein (Flow (GCV)) and coronary sinus (Flow (CS)) respectively:

CVR (GCV) = MAP/Flow(GCV) (mmHg · min/ml)

CVR (CS) = MAP/Flow(CS) (mmHg · min/ml)

Lactate Measurements

Blood (1.5 ml) for lactate measurements was rapidly deproteinized with an equal volume of cold 8% perchloric acid ($HClO_4$) and centrifuged. After centrifugation, the supernatant fluids were stored at $-20\,°C$. Lactate in the supernatant was analyzed enzymatically according to Apstein et al. [10] with the AutoAnalyzer. Standard curves were made with lithium lactate in 4% $HClO_4$.

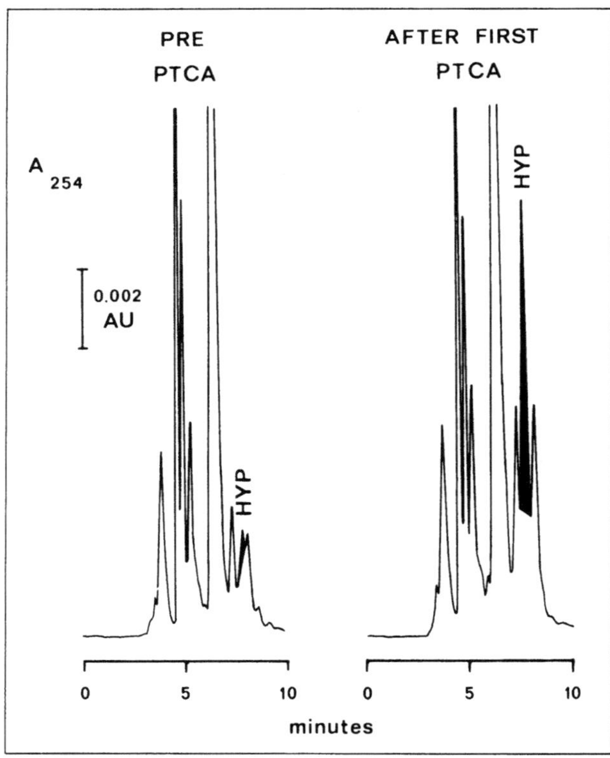

Fig. 1. Isocratic high-pressure liquid chromatographic separation of nucleosides and purine basis from a patient before and after a single transluminal occlusion. hyp, Hypoxanthine

An isocratic high-pressure liquid chromatographic system was used for the estimation of purine nucleosides and oxypurines in blood [11] (Fig. 1). Use was made of a reversed-phase column. Since nucleotides derived from erythrocytes affected the separation, these compounds had to be removed. We used the method of Chatterjee et al. [12], with some minor differences.

Blood samples were obtained at six consecutive measurement periods: before the PTCA procedure, 5-10 s after each transluminal occlusion, and 5 min after termination of the PTCA procedure. Five minutes were allowed between each dilatation for recovery.

Results are given either as mean ± standard deviation or as median values. Comparisons between pre-PTCA, post-PTCA, and 20-s and 50-s occlusion conditions were performed using two-way analysis of variance with orthogonal contrast.

Comparisons between pre-PTCA, post-PTCA, and occlusion conditions were evaluated using analysis of variance for repeated measurements. When overall significance was found, multiple comparisons were significantly different at the 0.05 level.

Table 1. Hemodynamic variables before PTCA, at 20 and 50 s after occlusion, and after the PTCA procedure

	pre-PTCA		20-s occlusion	50-s occlusion	post-PTCA	
	Total group (n = 14)	Subgroup (n = 9)	Total group (n = 14)	Subgroup (n = 9)	Subgroup (n = 9)	Total group (n = 14)
HR, bpm	62 ± 16	59 ± 18	61 ± 13	62 ± 14	63 ± 11	64 ± 11
EDVI, ml/m²	81 ± 15	79 ± 14	81 ± 15	81 ± 16	78 ± 11	77 ± 11
ESVI, ml/m²	31 ± 9	29 ± 7	$37 \pm 9*$	$41 \pm 9*$	26 ± 15	$27 \pm 7°$
SVI, ml/m²	50 ± 11	49 ± 11	$44 \pm 12°$	$39 \pm 14°$	52 ± 10	50 ± 9
EF, %	61 ± 8	62 ± 6	$54 \pm 8*$	$48 \pm 12*$	66 ± 6	64 ± 7
peak LVP, mmHg	154 ± 30	151 ± 35	142 ± 29	145 ± 37	148 ± 25	147 ± 21
peak dP/dt, mmHg · s⁻¹	1403 ± 304	1356 ± 257	1312 ± 320	1278 ± 317	1442 ± 284	1412 ± 333
V_{max}, s⁻¹	39 ± 9	40 ± 8	39 ± 9	$34 \pm 10°$	43 ± 12	42 ± 11
ESP, mmHG	95 ± 18	92 ± 22	90 ± 19	98 ± 24	91 ± 15	90 ± 14
Peak −dP/dt, mmHg · s⁻¹	1727 ± 322	1614 ± 267	$1268 \pm 355*$	$1404 \pm 370°$	1665 ± 296	1664 ± 243
Tau₁, ms	55 ± 8	55 ± 6	$79 \pm 17*$	$68 \pm 16*$	56 ± 7.5	54 ± 7
Tau₂, ms	44 ± 7	43 ± 7	$51 \pm 8°$	$59 \pm 8*$	45 ± 8	45 ± 9
P_{min}, mmHG	10 ± 5	8 ± 3	11 ± 4	$16 \pm 6*$	8 ± 5	8 ± 4
EDP, mmHG	22 ± 8	18 ± 6	22 ± 7	$29 \pm 5*$	21 ± 5	20 ± 6

Abbreviations: **PTCA,** percutaneous transluminal coronary angioplasty; **HR,** heart reate, **bpm,** beats per minute; **EDVI,** dend-diastolic volume index; **ESVI,** end-systolic volume index; **SVI,** stroke volume index; **EF,** ejection fraction; **LVP,** left ventricular pressure; **dP/dt,** rate of change of pressure; V_{max}, maximal velocity of the contractile element (dP/dt/P linearly extrapolated to P=O); **ESP,** end-systolic pressure; **Tau,** time constant of relaxation; **P_{min},** left ventricular minimal diastolic pressure; **EDP,** left ventricular end-diastolic pressure ° P < 0.05 compared with before PTCA, Student's paired t-test, * p < 0.005 compared with before PTCA

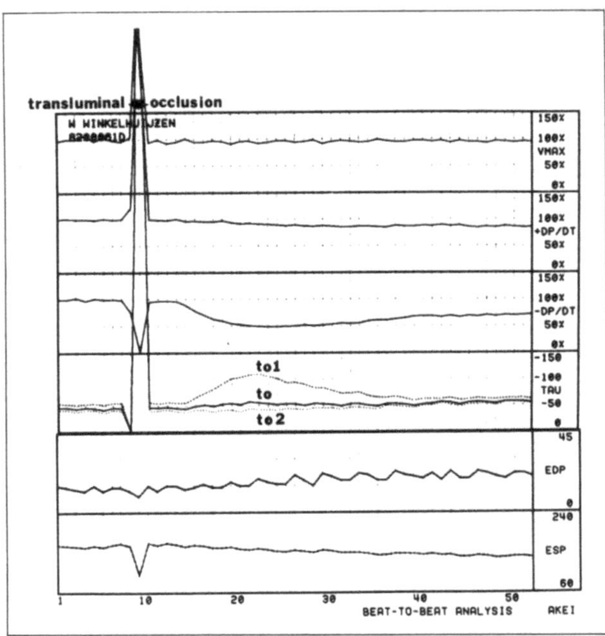

Fig. 2. Hemodynamic measurements in a patient during percutaneous transluminal coronary angioplasty. From **top** to **bottom**: maximal velocity of the contractile elements (V_{max}); peak ± and $-dP/dt$ expressed as a percentage of control values; the time constants of relaxation to_1 (dashed line), to (solid line), to_2 (dotted line) (scale 50 ms); end-diastolic pressure (**EDP**, scale 15 mmHg); peak systolic pressure (**ESP**, scale 60 mmHg, with 60 mmHg offset). The break in the data at beat 10 corresponds to inflation of the PTCA balloon

Results

Global Left Ventricular Function During Systole and Diastole

The left ventricular pressures and volumes measured before, during, and after angioplasty are shown in Table 1. There was no important change in heart rate during the PTCA procedure. The pattern of change in peak LVP, LVEDP, peak + dP/dt, and V_{max}, however, suggests a progressive depression in myocardial mechanics without any indication of an early peak (Fig. 2).

In contrast, within four or five beats after occlusion, a deformation appeared in the ascending limb of the negative dP/dt curve (Fig. 3), and in the next 10 s this deformation in the negative dP/dt curve gradually increased, so that the irregularity in the negative dP/dt curve reached the same height as peak −dP/dt which had progressively decreased to its nadir. In the next 20-50 s, peak −dP/dt began to return to control levels, with a resolution of the irregularity in the ascending limb of −dP/dt. At 50 s, peak −dP/dt recovered to 77% of the preocclusion value and the deformity was no longer present.

This deformation of the negative dP/dt signal at the early phase of the occlusion means that the time course of left ventricular pressure decay deviates substantially from the mono-exponential model usually proposed; it also means that asynchronous contraction or relaxation may be involved at the very beginning of the transluminal occlusion. Therefore, bi-exponential fitting of the pressure curve was computed during the isovolumic relaxation, primarily on the basis that, when plotted on semilogarithmic paper, the pressure curve was noted to follow two straight lines rather than the one predicted by the mono-exponential mode.

40

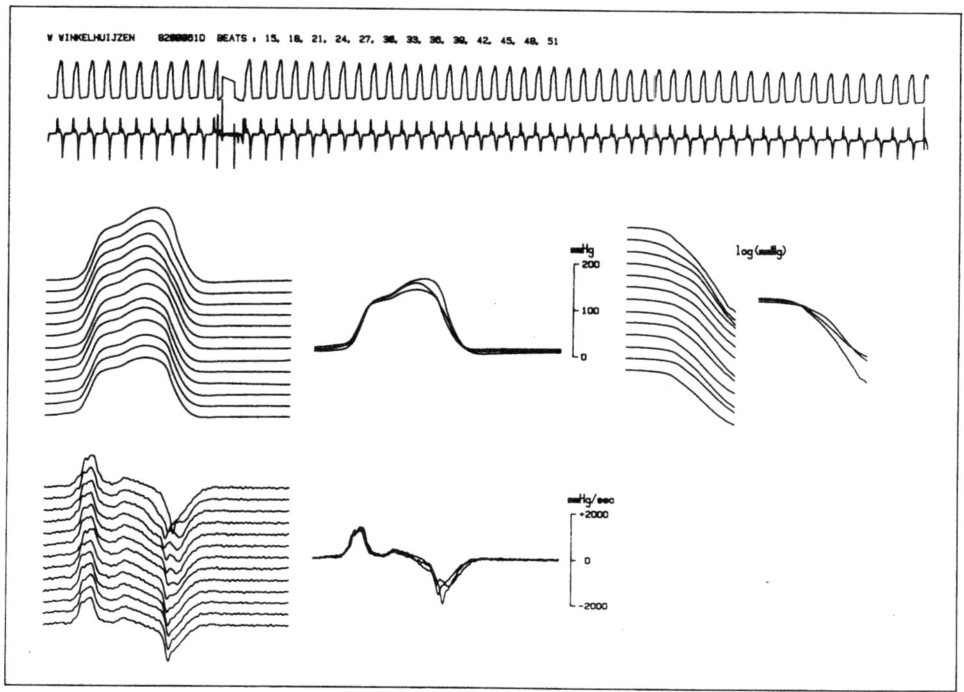

Fig. 3. Effects of coronary artery occlusion on left ventricular pressure (**mmHg**) and + and −dP/dt (**mmHg/sec**). The break in the recording at beat 15 corresponds to inflation of the balloon. On the **left hand side** are displayed the left ventricular pessure and + and −dP/dt of individual beats (15, 18, 21, and so forth), while the natural logarithm of the pressure is shown on the **right hand side**. Notice decrease in −dP/dt associated with an irregularity in the upstroke of the negative dP/dt curve. After 30 s (beat 42) peak −dP/dt starts to return toward a more normal shape of the signal

The second half of Table 1 summarizes the results of the relaxation parameters. The behavior of the two time constants (T_1, T_2) during PTCA is illustrated in Fig. 4.

The occlusion of a major coronary artery for 20 s resulted in a significant ($P < 0.005$) increase in end-systolic volume (from 31 ± 9 to 38 ± 9 ml/m²), while the end-diastolic volume remained unchanged after 20 s and even after 50 s of transluminal occlusion.

At 50 s, the ejection fraction decreased from 62% to 48% ($P\ 0.005$), and this decrease was essentially due to an increase in end-systolic volume from 29 ± 7 to 41 ± 9 ml/m² ($P < 0.005$).

The relationship between left ventricular diastolic pressure and volume during transluminal occlusion is illustrated by one example (Fig. 6). It is evident that the entire diastolic pressure-volume relationship during transluminal occlusion is gradually shifted upward and to the right, so that at any given volume diastolic pressure was higher. This effect was consistently observed after 50 s of occlusion.

The hemodynamic and cineangiographic investigations performed after completion of the PTCA procedure demonstrated the perfect reversibility of the systolic function as well as the normalization of the different pressure-derived indices.

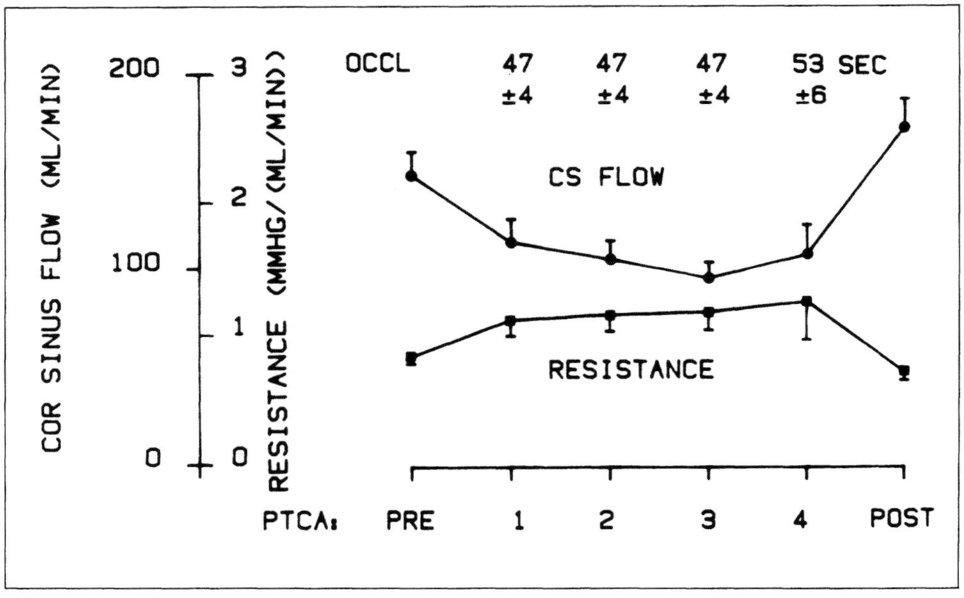

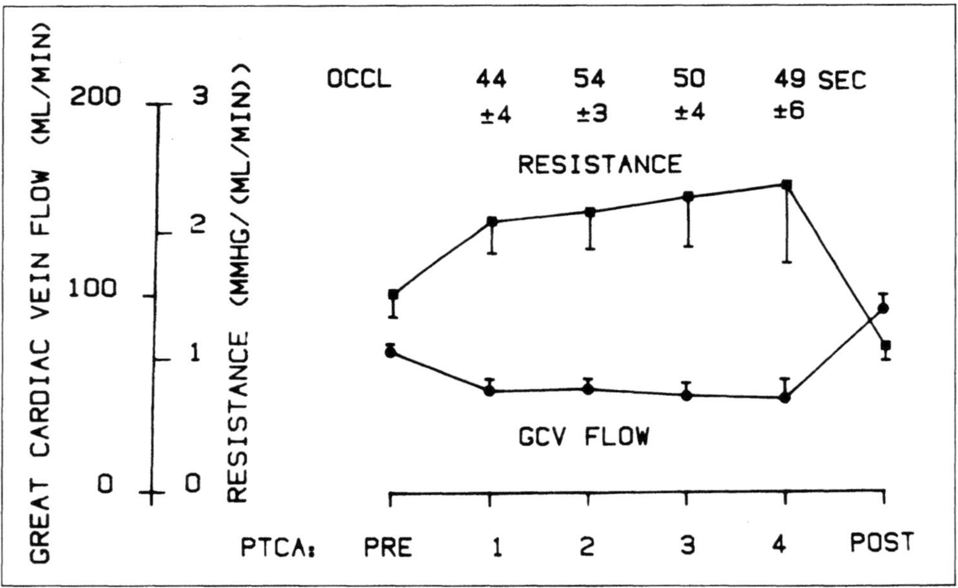

Fig. 4a. Changes in coronary sinus blood flow (ml/min) and resistance (mmHg/ml/min) during four episodes of occlusion. **CS**, coronary sinus. **b** Changes in great cardiac vein flow (ml/min) and resistance (mmHg/ml/min) during four transluminal occlusions. **occl**, occlusion time (s); **GCV**, great cardiac vein

The results of the coronary hemodynamic observations are summarized in Fig. 4. During the initial dilatation the mean duration of balloon inflation was 47 ± 4 s in group I and 44 ± 4 s in group II. During the subsequent dilatations the duration of inflation was slightly increased, up to 53 ± 6 s and 49 ± 6 s respectively. Occlusion pressure did not change throughout these occlusion times of 40-60s, and there was a high degree of reproducibility of the occlusion pressure during these successive occlusions. Coronary sinus blood flow before the first dilatation was 149 ± 12 ml/min, following to 96 ± 8 ml/min ($P < 0.005$) during the third transluminal occlusions and rising to 174 ± 15 ml/min (NS) 5 min after the last balloon deflation. Consequently, total coronary resistance increased from 0.75 ± 0.06 to 1.2 ± 0.3 mmHg/ml/min ($P < 0.05$) by the end of the fourth dilatation (Table 2).

The mean blood flow in the great cardiac vein in group II before the first inflation was 72 ± 4 ml/min, falling to 47 ± 10 ml/min (P 0.003) during the fourth inflation and rising slightly to 93 ± 8 ml/min ($P < 0.03$) after completion of the PTCA procedure, while the differences in resting pre- and post-coronary angioplasty levels of coronary sinus blood flow did not reach a statistically significant level. Great cardiac vein coronary vascular resistance was 1.42 ± 0.18 mmHg/min/ml before balloon inflation, 2.3 ± 0.6 by the end of the fourth inflation ($P < 0.005$), and 1.02 ± 0.11 after completion of the PTCA procedure (Table 3).

Table 2. Coronary hemodynamics and metabolic disturbances during sequential transluminal occlusion in group **I** (13 patients) procedure

	Before PTCA	First occlusion	Second occlusion	Third occlusion	Fourth occlusion	After PTCA
Duration of occlusion (s)	–	47 ± 4*	47 ± 4	47 ± 4	53 ± 6	–
Occlusion pressure (mmHg)	–	31 ± 5	28 ± 5	29 ± 3	30 ± 5	
CS flow (ml/min)	149 ± 12	115 ± 12^b	106 ± 9^b	96 ± 8^b	108 ± 15^a	174 ± 15
Resistance (mmHg/ml/min)	0.75 ± 0.06	1.03 ± 0.12^a	1.07 ± 0.13^a	1.09 ± 0.14^a	1.2 ± 0.3^a	0.64 ± 0.07
Arterial lactate (mM)	0.43 ± 0.09	0.46 ± 0.08	0.47 ± 0.09	0.43 ± 0.06	0.42 ± 0.06	0.42 ± 0.12
CS venous lactate (mM)	0.47 ± 0.10	0.81 ± 0.16^a	0.88 ± 0.19^b	0.75 ± 0.14^b	0.79 ± 0.14^a	0.46 ± 0.07
Art-CS lactate (mM)	-0.04 ± 0.04	-0.39 ± 0.14^a	-0.41 ± 0.14^a	-0.32 ± 0.08^b	-0.37 ± 0.10^b	-0.01 ± 0.07
Arterial hypoxanthine (μM)	1.81 ± 0.5	2.5 ± 1.1	1.9 ± 0.6	1.3 ± 0.4	1.6 ± 0.5	1.6 ± 0.5
CS venous hypoxanthine (μM)	2.2 ± 0.6	4.6 ± 1.4^a	3.0 ± 0.3	2.9 ± 0.9	2.5 ± 0.5	1.9 ± 0.3
Art-CS hypoxanthine (μM)	-0.4 ± 0.2	-2.04 ± 1.3	-0.9 ± 0.5	-1.7 ± 1.0	-0.9 ± 0.6	-0.1 ± 0.4

CS, coronary sinus; Art, arterial

*Mean $\pm$ SEM

[a] $p > .05$; [b] $p > .005$ versus before PTCA

Table 3. Coronary hemodynamics and metabolic disturbances during sequential transluminal occlusion in group **II** (15 patients)

	Before PTCA	First occlusion	Second occlusion	Third occlusion	Fourth occlusion	After PTCA
Duration of occlusion	–	44 ± 4*	54 ± 3	50 ± 4	49 ± 6	–
Occlusion pressure (mmHg)	–	24 ± 4	23 ± 3	21 ± 2	25 ± 5	
GCV flow (ml/min)	72 ± 4	51 ± 6^a	52 ± 6^a	48 ± 7^b	47 ± 10^b	93 ± 8^a
Resistance (mmHg/ml/min)	1.42 ± 0.18	2.0 ± 0.3^a	2.1 ± 0.3^a	2.2 ± 0.4^b	2.3 ± 0.6^b	1.02 ± 0.11
Arterial lactate (mM)	0.59 ± 0.12	0.67 ± 0.16	0.65 ± 0.12	0.71 ± 0.14	0.9 ± 0.3	0.58 ± 0.13
GCV lactate (mM)	0.75 ± 0.15	1.8 ± 0.4^b	1.6 ± 0.3^c	1.3 ± 0.3^b	1.8 ± 0.6^a	0.64 ± 0.12
Art-GCV lactate (mM)	-0.18 ± 0.06	-1.1 ± 0.3^a	-0.91 ± 0.18	-0.60 ± 0.17^b	-0.8 ± 0.4^b	-0.07 ± 0.03
Arterial hypoxanthine (μM)	3.0 ± 0.6	3.0 ± 0.7	3.3 ± 0.6	2.9 ± 0.8	3.0 ± 1.4	3.7 ± 0.7
GCV hypoxanthine (μM)	3.4 ± 0.7	5.2 ± 0.8^c	7.8 ± 1.4^b	4.2 ± 1.06	4.4 ± 1.2^a	3.8 ± 0.7
Art-GCV hypoxanthine (μM)	-0.3 ± 0.3	-2.2 ± 0.7^a	-4.52 ± 1.4^b	-1.4 ± 0.7	-1.5 ± 0.4	-0.2 ± 0.44

GCV, great cardiac vein; **Art,** = arterial; * Mean $\pm$ SEM
[a]p < .05; [b] p < .005; [c] p < .001 versus before PTCA

Lactate and Hypoxanthine Metabolism

The arteriovenous lactate measurements are shown in Fig. 5. In group II the control measurements showed a difference of -0.18 mM, which decreased to -1.1 and -0.91 mM after the first and the second dilatations respectively. After the third dilatation the lactate difference was -0.60 mM, which was not significantly different from the values recorded after the first and the second dilatations. As a first approximation, the amount of lactate lost from the ischemic tissue during the four consecutive occlusions seemed to be more or less constant and at least did not increase with the time. As expected, the pooled A-V lactate difference obtained during PTCA in group II (great cardiac vein, -0.8 ± 0.3 mM sampling) was higher than that in group I (coronary sinus sampling, -0.35 ± 0.12 mM/l ($P < 0.01$). During the four consecutive transluminal occlusions, an average rise in the great cardiac vein hypoxanthine from 3.4 ± 0.7 to 5.6 ± 1.1 μM ($P < 0.01$) and in coronary sinus hypoxanthine from 2.2 ± 0.6 to 3.6 ± 0.8 μM ($P < 0.05$) was observed, which fell off after completion of the PTCA procedure. The arterial levels of these compounds remained constant during transluminal occlusion. The myocardial arterial-GCV difference of hypoxanthine changed from -0.3 ± 0.3 μM before angioplasty at rest to -2.4 ± 1.2 μM (P 0.01) during sequential transluminal occlusions; this was significantly larger than the changes observed in the myocardial arterial-CS difference. Significant production of hypoxanthine, calculated either as arterial-venous difference or extraction, took place only during transluminal occlusion, while hypoxanthine release was absent 5 min after completion of the PTCA procedure.

44

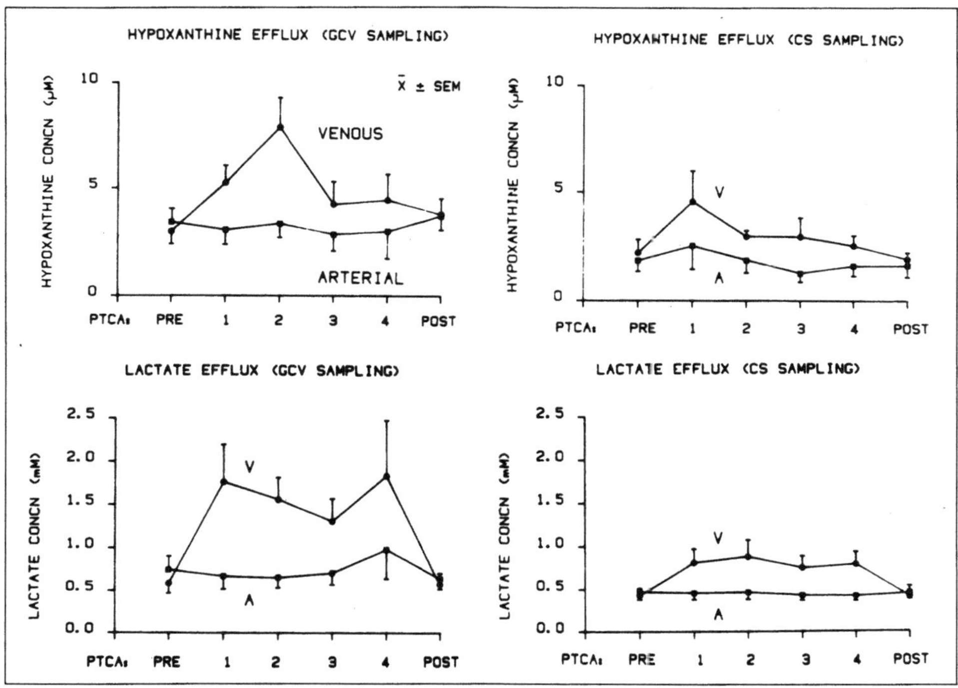

Fig. 5. Changes in arterial and venous concentration of hypoxanthine and lactate during transluminal occlusion. **GCV,** great cardiac vein; **CS,** coronary sinus; **pre,** pre-angioplasty; **post,** post-angioplasty

The crucial conclusion to be drawn from the observation that a few minutes after termination of the procedure no significant amount of lactate and hypoxanthine are produced is that metabolic disturbances induced by repeated ischemia are quickly reversible.

Discussion

Global and Regional Left Ventricular Performance

The earliest (1-15 s after occlusion) and most sensitive hemodynamic indicator of regional perfusion deficit proved to be an impairment in early relaxation, with extreme prolongation of T_1, the time constant of the early relaxation phase. If the premise of the two time-constant models previously described [7] is correct, then the early change in T_1 with a constant T_2 represents an exacerbation in the asynchrony of relaxation.
This is illustrated by the change in negative dP/dt and wall displacement induced by a 20-s coronary occlusion (Fig. 6). Within four or five beats after occlusion, a distinct deformation appears in the ascending limb of the negative dP/dt curve, and in the next 10 s this deformation reaches the same height as peak −dP/dt, which in the meantime has pro-

gressively decreased to its nadir. Accompanying this change in negative dP/dt, the ischemic segments exhibit a biphasic inward-outward wall displacement that occurs after valve closure and peak negative dP/dt. During the remainder of relaxation and rapid filling the ischemic segments display a second wave of inward wall displacement. The beginning of this second wave of inward wall displacement in early diastole corresponds closely in time to the irregularity in dP/dt. In the same way, the peak inward displacement of the control segment is consistently observed near the notching in the dP/dt. Shortly after this point, the pressure ceases to have a relaxation time constant T_1 and abruptly switches to T_2. On the other hand, after 50 s of occlusion the majority of the ischemic segments were akinetic, exhibiting an increased regional stiffness, whereas T_1, the time constant of the early relaxation phase, tended to return to less abnormal values. At 50 s the deformity in $-dP/dt$ was no longer present.

The connection between transient asynergy, myocardial ischemia, and alteration in the time course of relaxation was pointed out as early as 1969 by Tyberg et al. [13], who designed an experimental model consisting of two papillary muscles in series; they demonstrated that when one muscle of the pair was hypoxic, but still contracting, it was disturbing the time course of the total tension fall generated by the two muscles much more than when one of the muscles in series was not contracting at all and infinitely stiff [13]. More recent studies in conscious animals after experimental coronary occlusion have indicated that ventricular dyssynchrony due to late systolic contraction and relaxa-

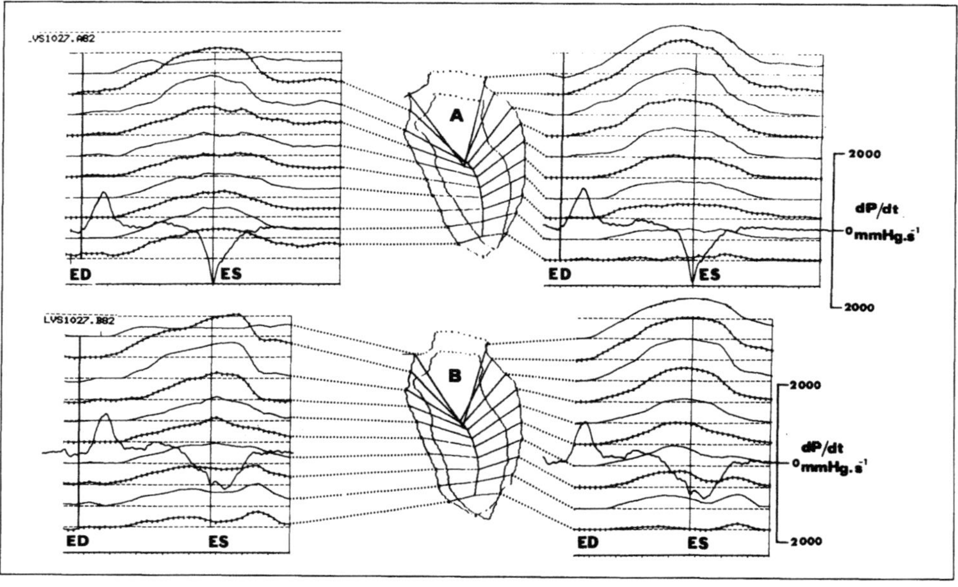

Fig. 6. Left ventricular wall displacement studied in 20 separate segments, ten in the anterior (**right**) and ten in the inferoposterior wall (**left**). A typical example of the relation between segmental wall displacement and dP/dt curve is observed before PTCA (**A**) and after 20 s (**B**) of left anterior descending artery occlusion: after 20 s of occlusion, the notch in the dP/dt curve corresponds to a second wave of inward wall displacement in the antero- and inferoapical segments

tion in different regions can produce marked effects on the linearity and maximal rate of pressure fall in the left ventricle [14-16].

The present study suggests that a similar phenomenon may occur in the intact human heart during acute ischemia. At 20 s, the late systolic outward displacement of the ischemic segment is probably passive and is due to a simultaneously segments. Conversely, the early diastolic inward displacement of the ischemic segments must correspond to an accelerated outward displacement of the normal segment. Ultimately, after 20 s of ischemia the ischemic zone appears to act as an additional elastic element, in series with the actively contracting and relaxing nonischemic segment. This mechanism is consistent with the model of LV pressure relaxation recently proposed by our group [7], which assumes that the observed time constant T1 results from the combined action of that fraction of the myocardium in the process of relaxing and the remainder yet to initiate relaxation.

Use of Purine Release as a Marker for Ischemia During Transluminal Occlusion in Man

Ischemia can be defined as a situation in which coronary blood flow (and hence oxygen and substrate supply, and carbon dioxide and metabolite removal) cannot meet the tissue demand [17]. As a consequence of this O_2 deficiency, mitochondrial function is restricted [18], and the balance between ATP production and usage is disturbed; creatine phosphate (CrP) levels fall, followed by a decline in ATP [19]. Creatine (Cr), ADP, phosphate and H^+ levels increase [20-22], the glycolysis rate is increased [23, 24], and lactate levels rise. Shortly thereafter, K^+, H^+, and lactate are released into the coronary venous blood.

The anaerobic ATP production, however, is insufficient to meet the amount of ATP needed for contraction [21]. This is directly responsible for the decrease in local segmental wall function [1, 25], which is in turn reflected by a loss of systolic wall thickening [1] and shortening [26].

If sufficiently widespread, global hemodynamic measurements will demonstrate a decrease in contractility as reflected by a decrease in LV ejection fraction, and in the maximal velocity of the contractile element (Vmax), as well as an increae in regional myocardial stiffness with a reduction in LV distensibility, which manifests itself by an increase in end-diastolic pressure [27, 28]. This series of events was repeatedly observed in our patients during transluminal angioplasty.

When ATP levels decrease, cellular ADP levels increase. ATP is converted to ADP and AMP by the action of adenylate kinase. AMP is deaminated to IMP, or dephosphorylated to adenosine, which is further catabolized to inosine and hypoxanthine (Fig. 7). These components pass the cell membrane [25, 29-31], where adenosine acts as a vasodilator [31, 32]. A slight decrease in ATP therefore results in an immediate rise in AMP catabolites. This release can be used to monitor myocardial ATP breakdown.

We felt therefore that measuring myocardial arterial-venous differences of blood hypoxanthine levels could give insight into the metabolic state of the heart; the method used here makes it possible to measure a number of purine metabolites in blood. A close correlation has been found between purine and lactate release from animal and human hearts [11, 33-39]. As a marker of ischemia, however, lactate has several disadvantages. During normoxia, lactate is preferentially taken up by the heart [40]. In fact, lactate released from a local ischemic area can be metabolized by the surrounding normoxic tissue

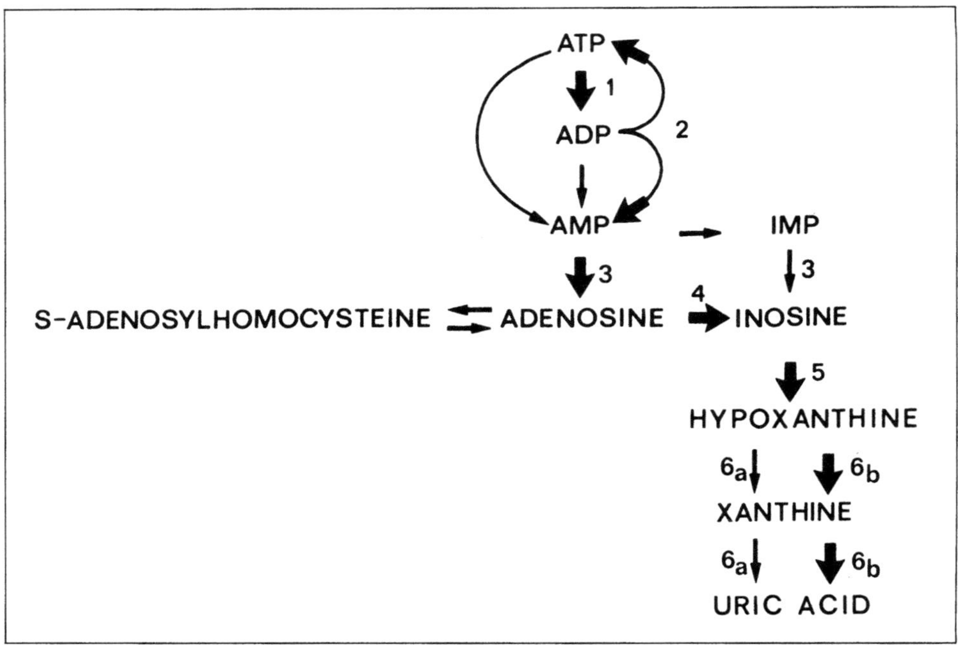

Fig. 7. Myocardial ATP catabolism. The main pathways are: **1,** ATPase; **2,** adenylate kinase; **3,** 5'-nucleotidase; **4,** adenosine deaminase; **5,** nucleoside phosphorylase; **6a,** xanthine oxidase; **6b,** xanthine dehydrogenase

[23]. The formation and removal of lactate is also influenced by blood fatty acid levels, acidosis, and by hyperglycemia [41], all metabolic conditions likely to be present during angioplasty. In addition, observations on the patients undergoing an atrial pacing stress test indicate that hypoxanthine is a more sensitive parameter for myocarial ischemia than adenosine, inosine, xanthine, or lactate, because hypoxanthine release is more pronounced and of a longer duration than that of the other compounds [11].

Since we could not record the great cardiac vein or coronary sinus flow during the sampling period, we did not express our results in terms of lactate or hypoxanthine efflux. The less elevated concentrations of lactate and hypoxanthine in the great cardiac vein after the third sequential occlusion do not necessarily reflect a reduction in lactate or hypoxanthine production, since the reactive hyperemia measured after the third occlusion might have been significantly greater than that measured after the first and second occlusions [27, 42]. Therefore, and as a first approximation, the amount of lactate and hypoxanthine lost from the ischemic tissue during the first two occlusions seems to be more or less constant and at least does not increase with sequential occlusions.

Previous work [43, 44] indicates that repetitive episodes of brief ischemia do not produce a cumulative depletion of high-energy phosphate compounds. The content of nucleotide pools at any point in time is determined by the rate of synthesis versus demand. The failure to demonstrate a progressive decrease in nucleotide pools during subsequent ischemic episodes following an initial ischemic episode might be explained by a decreased degradation of nucleotides during the subsequent ischemic episodes. Decreased degradation without increased synthesis is supported by the finding of the current study that the efflux of nucleotide catabolites (such as hypoxanthine) during reperfusion after the third or the fourth occlusion was less than, or at least not significantly different from the values obtained after the first or the second coronary occlusion.

The mechanism for the decrease in coronary nucleotide degradation during subsequent episodes of ischemia is unclear, but several explanations can be proposed to account for this finding. There is growing evidence for compartmentation of myocardial nucleotide pools [45, 46]. The different compartments in the cell may have different susceptibilities to depletion during myocardial ischemia. Susceptible pools may be depleted during the first ischemic episode, with more resistant pools remaining intact during subsequent ischemic episodes of the same duration. Another which may have contributed to the reduction in nucleotide degradation during the second and third occlusion is the greater than normal CrP content of myocardium following a brief ischemic episode [47, 48].

Whatever the mechanism, the increased stores presumably present at the onset of the second and third coronary occlusions may provide high-energy phosphate which serves to protect ATP pools from further depletion. A third potential explanation for decreased nucelotide degradation during the ischemic period is decreased energy consumption from decreased contractile function. However, even from the current hemodynamic study, it seems unlikely that more rapid contractile failure may account for the preservation of nucleotide pools observed during the third and fourth occlusions. Other hemodynamic factors have to be considered.

Rentrop et al. [49] have demonstrated during balloon inflation the angiographic appearance of a previously absent coronary collateral circulation. This apparent recruitment of collaterals might play a major role in the modulation of the ischemic and metabolic phenomenon related to the angioplasty procedure, although its functional significance is not yet well defined. It has been shown that the occlusion pressure measured distal to the stenosis during balloon inflation correlates well with the existence of a collateral circulation angiographically demonstrable before or during angioplasty [50, 51]. However, Probst et al. [50], Meier et al. [51], and we, ourselves, did not observe any change in the coronary occlusion pressure during serial occlusion. In fact, our results confirm their observations. The absence of any increase in coronary sinus and great cardiac vein flow during serial occlusions precludes the gradual recruitment of collateral circulation during repeated occlusions, which might have explained a progressive decrease in lactate and hypoxanthine efflux.

Metabolism During Reperfusion

The crucial conclusion to be drawn from our observations is that metabolic disturbances induced by repeated ischemia are quickly reversible, provided they are of short (<90 s) duration. During reperfusion, cells are reoxygenated and waste products removed. After ischemia, for a short period of time, reperfusion induces an enhanced Ca^{2+} influx, mitochondria are reactivated, and ATP and CrP are again produced [52, 53]. The latter compound is transported to the myofibrils. Because of ionogenic disturbances in the cell, contraction is still decreased at this stage, probably due to disturbed Ca2+ concentrations in the cell [54]. This can be demonstrated by an increased ventricular wall tension [55,

56], indicating an increased Ca^{2+} level, and an increased CrP, even to levels higher than the normal range [57]. This indicates that ATP consumption by contraction is at this state below ATP production. After activation of the ionic pumps, cellular homeostasis is restored and the cell starts beating again. However, ATP levels will remain subnormal for some time, and these low ATP levels cause an extra risk, inasmuch as a critically low ATP level will be reached earlier during the next ischemic attack [58, 59]. It was recently demonstrated that in isolated working rat hearts the early restoration of oxidative metabolism during reperfusion determines functional recovery of the reperfused ischemic myocardium, despite the presence of low ATP levels [60]. Thus, it seems that the integrity of the pathways of oxidative metabolism, rather than steady state ATP levels, plays a major role in the myocardial functional recovery after acute ischemia. Even so, the decline of high-energy phosphate stores heralds the beginning of "no return".

Clinical Implications

Experimental data on atherosclerotic vessel segments have shown that volume reduction of atherosclerotic tissue is related to the duration of pressure application. These findings have led many clinicians to use longer inflation durations (30-60 s) during PTCA [61, 62]. On the other hand, Braunwald an Kloner [58] have recently addressed the question of whether the myocardium can become chronically, even permanently "stunned" as a consequence of repetitive episodes of myocardial ischemia. Although most episodes of transient ischemia occurring in our patients during transluminal angioplasty are not as severe as those of the animal studies [16, 63, 64], the total duration of occlusive episodes during PTCA has increased considerably since our initial experience: the median is now 4 min, and a few cases exceed 10 min in our laboratory [2]. This total occlusion time of 4 min might be excessive, since it has been demonstrated in conscious dogs that the return of myocardial function is delayed after periods of coronary occlusion as brief as 100 s. Here, the reactive hyperemia which occurs normally during reperfusion is prevented by a residual subtotal occlusion [15], a situation which does not apply after successful PTCA. In this respect, the results of the present study seem to be reassuring, since there is no evidence of global or regional myocardial dysfunction even after four to six coronary occlusions, each of them lasting for 40-60 s.
Further work is needed to document the responsible derangements of subcellular metabollism, as the mechanisms of the observed abnormalities are not yet fully understood. Although recovery in terms of lactate and hypoxanthine metabolism is demonstrated, the question must remain as to what extent transport mechanisms and enzymatic reactions have been transiently altered.

References

1. Das SK, Serruys PW, van den Brand M, Domenicucci S, Vletter WB, Roelandt J (1983) Acute echocardiographic changes during percutaneous coronary angioplasty and their relationship to coronary blood flow. J Cardiovasc Ultrasonography 2: 269-271
2. Serruys PW, van den Brand M, Brower RW, Hugenholtz PG (1983) Regional cardioplegia and cardioprotection during transluminal angioplasty, which role for nifedipine? Eur Heart J 4: 115–121

3. Meester GT, Bernard N, Zeelenberg C, Brower RW, Hugenholtz PG (1975) A computer system for real-time analysis of cardiac catheterization data. Cathet Cardiovasc Diagn 1: 112-123

4. Meester GT, Zeelenberg C, Bernard N, Gorter S (1974) Beat-to-beat analysis of cardiac catheterization data. In: Computers in cardiology. IEEE Computer Society, Los Angeles, pp 63-65

5. Thompson DS, Waldron CB, Juul SM, Naqvi N, Swanton RH, Coltart DJ, Jenkins BS, Webb-Peploe MM (1982) Analysis of left ventricular pressure during isovolumic relaxation in coronary artery disease. Circulation 65: 690-697

6. Bernardi L, Uretsky BF, Reddy PS, Boudreau R (1985) Modeling the isovolumic relaxation period. Cathet Cardiovasc Diagn 11: 255-268

7. Brower RW, Meij S, Serruys PW (1983) A model of asynchronous left ventricular relaxation predicting the bi-exponential pressure decay. Cardiovasc Res 17: 482-488

8. Slager CJ, Reiber JHC, Schuurbiers JCH, Meester GT (1978) Contouromat – a hard-wired left ventricular angio processing system. Design and application. Comput Biomed Res 11: 491-502

9. Metha, J, Pepine CJ (1978) Effect of sublingual nitroglycerin on regional flow in patients with and without coronary disease. Circulation 58: 803-807

10. Apstein CS, Puchner E, Brachfeld N (1979) Improved automated lactate determination. Anal Biochem 38: 20-34

11. Harmsen E, de Jong JW, Serruys PW (1981) Hypoxanthine production by ischemic heart demonstrated by high-pressure liquid chromatography of blood purine nucleosides and oxypurines. Clin Chim Acta 115: 73-84

12. Chatterjee SK, Bhattacharya M, Barlow JJ (1979) A simple, specific radiometric assay for 5'-nucleotides. Anal Biochem 95: 497-506

13. Tyberg JV, Parmley WW, Sonnenblick EH (1986) In vitro studies of myocardial asynchrony and regional hypoxia. Circ Res 25: 569-579

14. Kumada T, Karliner JS, Pouleyr H, Gallagher KP, Shirato K, Ross J jr (1979) Effects of coronary occlusion on early ventricular diastolic events in conscious dogs. Am J Physiol 237: H542-H549

15. Pagani M, Vatner SF, Baig H, Braunwald E (1978) Initial myocardial adjustment to brief periods of ischema and reperfusion in the conscious dog. Cir Res 43 (1): 83-92

16. Theroux P, Ross J jr, Franklin D, Kemper WS, Sasayama S (1976) Regional myocardial function in the conscious dog during acute coronary occlusion and responses to morphine, propanolol, nitroglycerine and lidocaine. Circulation 53: 302-314

17. Manning AS, Hearse DJ, Dennis SC, Bullock GR, Coltard DJ (1980) Myocardial ischemia: an isolated, globally perfused rat heart model for metabolic and pharmacological studies. Eur J Cardiol 11: 1-21

18. Wilson DF, Owen CS, Erecinska M (1979) Quantitative dependence of mitochondrial oxidative phosphorylation on oxygen concentration. A new mathematical model. Arch Biochem Biophys 195: 494-504

19. de Jong JW (1979) Biochemistry of acutely ischemic myocardium. In: Schaper W (ed) The pathophysiology of myocardial perfusion. Elsevier/North-Holland, Amsterdam, pp 719-750

20. Garlick BP, Radda GK, Seeley PJ (1979) Studies of acidosis in the ischaemic heart by pohsphorus nuclear magnetic resonance. Biochem J 184: 547-554

21. Hearse DJ (1979) Oxygen deprivation and early myocardial contractile failure. Reassessment of the possible role of adenosine triphosphate. Am J Cardiol 44: 1115-1120

22. Hearse DJ, Drome R, Yellon DM, Wyse R (1983) Metabolic and flow correlates of myocardial ischemia. Cardiovasc Res 17: 452-458

23. Apstein CS, Deckelbaum L, Mueller M, Hagopian L, Hood WB (1977) Graded global ischemia and reperfusion. Circulation 55: 864-872

24. Neely JR, Liedke AJ, Whitmer TJ, Rovetto MJ (1975) Relationship between coronary flow and adenosine triphosphate production from glycolysis and oxidative metabolism. Recent Adv Studies Cardiac Structure Metab 8: 301-321

25. de Jong JW, Goldstein S (1974) Changes in coronary venous inosine concentration and myocardial wall thickening during regional ischemia in the pig. Circ. Res 35: 111-116

26. Jaski BE, Serruys PW (1985) Epicardial wall motion and left ventricular function during coronary graft angioplasty in humans. J Am Coll Cardiol 6: 695-700

27. Serruys PW, Wijns W, Grimm J, Slager C, Hess OM (1984) Effects of repeated transluminal occlusions during angioplasty on global and regional left ventricular chamber stiffness (abstr). Circulation 70 [Suppl II]: 348

28. Serruys PW, Wijns W, van den Brand M, et al. (1984) Left ventricular performance, regional blood flow, wall motion and lactate metabolism during transluminal angioplasty. Circulation 70: 25-36

29. de Boer LWV, Ingwall JS, Kloner RA, Braunwald E (1980) Prolonged derangements of canine myocardial purine metabolism after brief coronary artery occlusion not associated with anatomic evidence of necrosis. Proc Natl Acad Sci USA 77: 5471-5475

30. de Jong JW, Harmsen E, de Tombe PP, Keijzer E (1983) Release of purine nucleosides and oxypurines from the isolated perfused rat heart. Adv Myocardiol 4: 339-345

31. Schrader J, Haddy FJ, Gerlach E (1979) Release of adenosine, inosine and hypoxanthine from the isolated guinea pig heart during hypoxia, flow-autoregulation and reactive hyperemia. Pflugers Arch 369: 251-257

32. Berne RM (1980) The role of adenosine in the regulation of coronary blood flow. Circ Res 47: 807-813

33. Fox AC, Reed GE, Mellman H, Silk BB (1979) Release of nucleosides from canine and human hearts as an index of prior ischemia. Am J Cardiol 43: 52-57

34. Kugler G (1978) The effects of nitroglycerin on myocardial release of inosine, hypoxanthine and lactate during pacing induced angina. Basic Res Cardiol 73: 523-533

35. Kugler G (1979) Myocardial release of lactate, inosine and hypoxanthine during atrial pacing and exercise-induced angina. Circulation 59: 43-49

36. Brower RW, de Jong JW, Haalebos M, et al. (1982) Evaluation of cardioplegia in coronary artery bypass graft surgery. In Just H, Tschirkov A, Schlosser V (eds) Kalziumantagonisten zur Kardioplegie und Myocardprotection in der offenen Herzchirurgie. Thieme, Stuttgart, pp 69-80

37. Serruys PW, de Jong JW, Harmsen E, Verdouw PD, Hugenholtz PG (1983) Effect of intracoronary nifedipine in high-energy phosphate metabolism during repeated pacing-induced angina and during experimental ischemia. In: Kaltenbach M, Neufield HN (eds) New therapy of ischemic heart disease and hypertension. Excerpta Medica, Amsterdam, pp 340-353

38. Edlund A, Berglund B, van Dorne D, et al. (1985) Coronary flow regulation in patients with ischemic heart disease: release of purines and prostacyclin and the effect of inhibitors of prostaglandin formation. Circulation 6: 1113-1120

39. Schoenberg MH, Fredholm BB, Hohlbach G (1985) Changes in acid-base status, lactate concentration and purine metabolics during reconstructive aortic surgery. Acta Chir Scand 151: 227-233

40. Drake AJ, Haines JR, Noble MIM (1980) Preferential uptake of lactate by the normal myocardium in dogs. Cardiovasc Res 14: 65-77

41. Verdouw PW, Stam H (1980) In: Moret PR et al. (eds) Lactate. Physiologic, methodologic and pathologic approach. Springer-Verlag, Berlin Heidelberg New York, pp 207-223

42. Rothman MT, Baim DS, Simpson JB, Harrison DC (1982) Coronary hemodynamics during percutaneous transluminal coronary angioplasty. Am J Cardiol 49: 1615-1621

43. Swain JL, Sabina RL, Hines JJ, Greenfield Jr JC, Holmes EW (1984) Repetitive episodes of brief ischemia (12 min) do not produce a cumulative depletion of high-energy phosphate compounds. Cardiovasc Res 18: 264-269

44. Verdouw PD, Remme WJ, de Jong JW, Breeman WAP (1979) Myocardial substrate utilization and hemodynamics following repeated coronary flow reduction in pigs. Basic Res Cardiol 74: 477-493

45. Gubdjarnason S, Mathes P, Revens KG (1970) Functional compartmentation of ATP and creatine phosphates in heart muscle. J Mol Cell Card 1: 325

46. Schrader J, Gerlach E (1976) Compartmentation of cardiac adenine nucleotides and formation of adenosine. Pflugers Arch 367: 129-135

47. Swain JL, Sabina RL, McHale PA, Greenfield JC jr, Holmes EW (1982) Prolonged myocardial nucleotide depletion after brief ischemia in the open-chest dog. Am J Physiol 242: H818-H826

48. Vial C, Font B, Goldschmidt D, Pearlman AS, Delaye J (1978) Regional myocardial energetics during brief periods of coronary occlusion and reperfusion: comparison with ST-segment changes. Cardiovasc Res 12: 470-476

49. Rentrop KP, Cohen M, Blanke H, Phillips RA (1985) Changes in collateral channel filling immediately after controlled coronary artery occlusion by an angioplasty balloon in human subjects. J Am Coll Cardiol 5: 587-592
50. Probst P, Zangl W, Pachinger O (1985) Relation of coronary arterial occlusion pressure during percutaneous transluminal coronary angioplasty to presence of collaterals. Am J Cardiol 55: 1264-1269
51. Meier B, Luethy P (1984) Coronary wedge pressure as predictor of recruitable collateral arteries. Circulation 70 [Suppl II]: 266
52. Hearse DJ (1977) Reperfusion of the ischemic myocardium (editorial). J Mol Cell Cardiol 9: 605-616
53. Mittnacht S, Sherman C, Farber JL (1981) Reversal of ischemic mitochondrial dysfunction. J Biol Chem 256: 3199-3206
54. Puri PS (1975) Contractile and biochemical effects of coronary reperfusion after extended periods of coronary occlusion. Am J Cardiol 36: 244-251
55. Apstein CS, Deckelbaum L, Hagopian L, Hood WB (1978) Acute cardiac ischemia and reperfusion: contractility, relaxation and glycolysis. Am J Physiol 235: H637-H648
56. Lewis MJ, Honsmand PR, Claes VA, Brutsaert DL, Henderson AH (1980) Myocardial stiffness during hypoxia and reoxygenation contracture. Cardiovasc Res 14: 339-344
57. Flaherty JT, Weisfeld ML, Buckley BH, Gardner TJ, Gott VT, Jacobus WE (1982) Mechanism of ischemic myocardial cell damage assessed by phosphorus-31 nuclear magnetic resonance. Circuluation 65: 561-576
58. Braunwald E, Kloner RA (1982) The "stunned" myocardium. Circulation 66: 1146-1149
59. Geft IL, Fishbein MC, Ninomiya K, et al (1982) Intermittent brief periods of ischemia have a cumulative effect and may cause myocardial necrosis. Circulation 66: 1150-1153
60. Taegtmeyer H, Roberts AFC, Raine AEG (1985) Emergency metabolism in reperfused heart muscle: metabolic correlates to return of function. J Am Coll Cardiol 6: 864-870
61. Schmitz HJ, Meyer J, Kiesslich T, Effert S (1982) Greater initial dilatation gives better late angiographic results in percutaneous coronary angioplasty (PTCA) Circulation 66 [Suppl II]: 62
62. Kaltenbach M, Kober G (1982) Can prolonged application of pressure improve the results of coronary angioplasty (PTCA)? Circulation 66 [Suppl II]: 123
63. Theroux P, Ross J jr, Franklin D, Covell JW, Bloor CM, Sasayama S (1977) Regional myocardial infarction in the unanesthetized dog. Circ Res 40: 158-165
64. Heijndrickx GR, Millard RW, McRitchie RJ, Maroko PR, Vatner SF (1975) Regional myocardial function and electrophysiological alterations after brief coronary artery occlusion in conscious dogs. J Clin Invest 56: 978-985

Author's adress:
Patrick W. Serruys, M.D.
Catheterization Laboratory
Thoraxcenter
P.O. Box 1738
3000 DR Rotterdam
The Netherlands

Selective Coronary Perfusion via Angioplasty Catheters – Technical and Physiological Aspects

U. W. Busch

I. Medizinische Klinik und Poliklinik rechts der Isar, München,
Federal Republic of Germany

Introduction

Transluminal coronary angioplasty has become an established form of treatment of coronary artery disease. Although Grüntzig initially suggested perfusion of the distal coronary artery with blood through the dilatation catheter during the procedure [1, 2], this has not become a routine part of the intervention. However, continuous selective coronary perfusion would possibly be used routinely under certain conditions if this could be accomplished in a safe and easy way, at least in cases with proximal stenosis of large, poorly collateralized vessels. It probably would be even more important in cases with dilatation-induced acute coronary occlusion, to prevent irreversible ischemic damage to the jeopardized myocardial area until surgical revascularization can be performed. With a large area at risk the danger of acute left ventricular failure and shock might be reduced or prevented if selective coronary perfusion could be of sufficient magnitude to maintain myocardial function.

The goal of our investigations was to evaluate possibilities of continuous selective coronary artery perfusion via angioplasty catheters in order to reduce or prevent myocardial ischemia during PTCA or following PTCA-induced acute coronary occlusion.

Methods and Results

Basically, continuous perfusion can be achieved in two ways: actively, with an external pump through the total length of the dilatation catheter after removal of the guide wire, or passively using a modified Grüntzig catheter that has side holes just proximal to the balloon, allowing blood to flow through the distal catheter segment by the existing transocclusional pressure gradient. Both ways have been evaluated in vitro and in animal experiments [3, 4].

Active Perfusion

For active perfusion through conventional dilatation catheters a special pump had to be developed that – unlike available roller pumps – provided sufficiently high pump pressures and flow rates, negligible mechanical hemolysis even at high pump pressures, reliable pump pressure and volume control, and AC independence for use during patient transfer. The technical solution was, in essence, a pneumatically driven, double-piston reciprocal pump, capable of producing pressures up to 15 atm and flow rates up to 160 ml/min.

During in vitro tests the pump pressure/flow rate relations were determined for various dilatation catheters in clinical use. In addition, the influence of perfusate viscosity was demonstrated, using full blood, Ringer's solution, and a 50 : 50 mixture of both. The results are shown in Fig. 1. Due to the larger internal lumen of the Grüntzig catheters over the whole length of the shaft proximal to the ballon, the pump pressure requirements for this type were of the order of 1/3-1/4 of the pressures needed with the Simpson-Robert catheter.

Despite these markedly increased pump pressures with the latter, however, hemolysis was not increased, as determined in vitro by measurement of total plasma hemoglobin rise during 30-min pumping of a recirculating blood pool of 100 ml at a rate of 60 ml/min. Excessively high hemolysis rates were found with the old, non-steerable Grüntzig catheters only, with all the blood leaving through the distal side-holes in a turbulent, jet-like fashion. Platelet count decreased to some extent with all catheters used, but, again, the most striking decrease was found with the old, non-steerable ones.

In vivo studies were carried out in 22 anesthetized, mechanically ventilated, closed-chest mongrel dogs. Prior to catheter insertion the animals were heparinized with an initial bolus of 10 000 U followed by subsequent infusion of 100 U/kg/h. In addition, ASA and

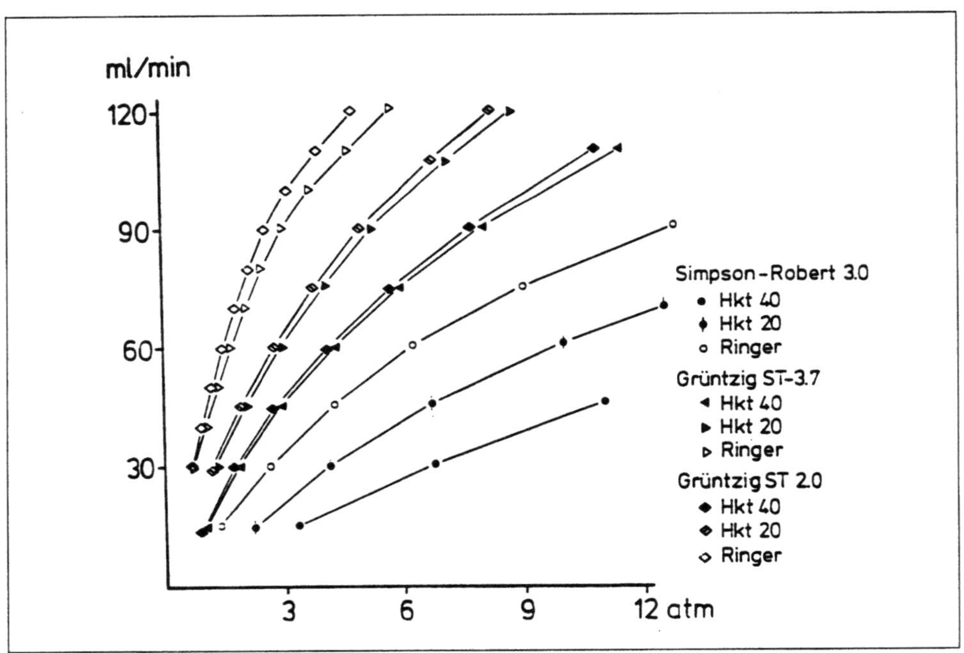

Fig. 1. Pressure/flow relations for perfusion through various coronary dilatation catheters with undiluted and diluted blood and Ringer's solution

dextran were given. Selective coronary perfusion with blood from the femoral artery through the angioplasty catheter was started after control measurements, and subsequent proximal balloon occlusion of either the LAD or LCx. The initial rate of 1 ml/min/kg body weight was increased if judged necessary by ECG and/or coronary venous O_2 saturation criteria suggestive of underperfusion, but maximally to 2.5 ml/min/kg body weight. Under stable conditions perfusion was performed over the intended 2-h period in 20 dogs; one dog died 4 min after balloon inflation from uncorrectable ventricular fibrillation, probably due to balloon occlusion of a larger septal perforator branch, and in another case there was thrombotic occlusion of the perfusion system after 35 min due to inadequate heparinization.

At the end of the 2-h period, terminating perfusion of the occluded coronary artery resulted in the development of marked ischemia in all but two dogs that probably had well – developed collateral circulation. In a few dogs with pre-existing ischemia (from balloon occlusion of side branches or inadequate perfusion rate in the presence of severe anemia) it led to a further increase of ischemic changes. Three dogs developed ventricular fibrillation within the first 7 min after perfusion was stopped. In ten dogs undergoing subsequent reperfusion at the previous rate ischemia-induced hemodynamic and ECG changes were fully reversible (see Fig. 2). Coronary venous O_2 saturation showed a gradual but constant rise during the 2-h perfusion period, a significant drop during non-perfusion, and a return to the preischemic level with reperfusion. In the individual case, however,

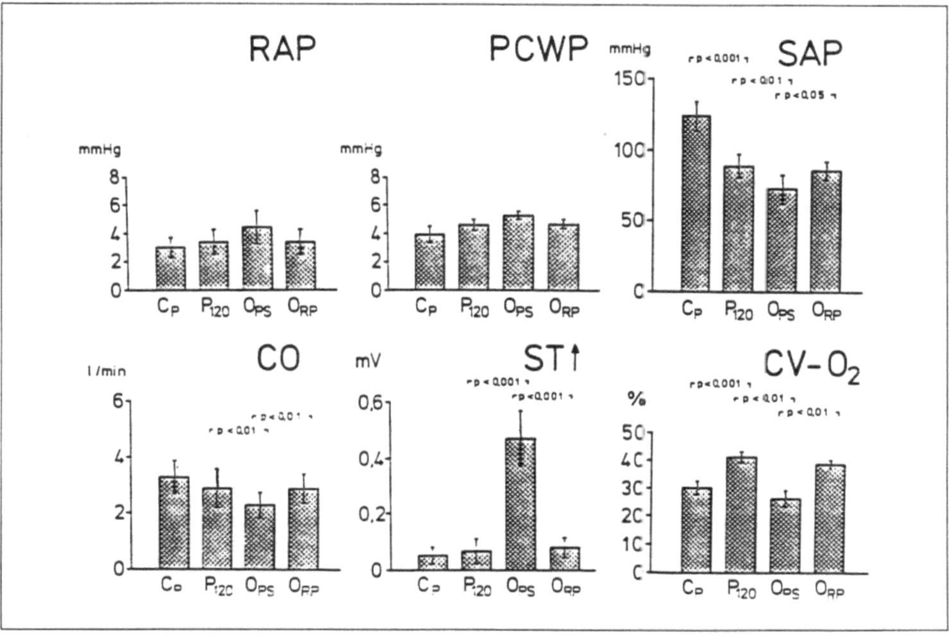

Fig. 2. Hemodynamic parameters, ST-segment changes, and coronary venous O_2 saturations during the perfusion experiment. C_p control; P120, at 120 min of selective perfusion of the proximally occluded coronary artery; OPS, after perfusion stop of the occluded artery; ORP with reperfusion

interruption of antegrade coronary blood flow did not necessarily result in a sustained or even transient fall in coronary venous O_2 saturation.

Intravascular pressure within the occluded vessel, measured through an additional, short perfusion catheter (2.5 F), never reached critically high values and varied between 61% and 120% of the actual aortic pressure. Even at a constant perfusion rate the intravascular pressure showed rather marked fluctuations during the 2-h perfusion period.

Passive Perfusion

During in vitro testing of the modified Grüntzig catheter (CPC catheter), the flow rates obtained with effective pressure gradients in the physiological range of 25–100 mmHg were between 18 and 44 ml/min for normal saline. For blood, flow rates were significantly lower and varied – depending upon blood viscosity, which is mainly determined by the hematocrit – between 6 and 12 ml/min at an effective pressure of 25 mmHg and between 21 and 32 ml/min at 100 mmHg (Fig. 3). Balloon filling pressures between 2 and 8 atm did not influence flow rate, indicating that there was no measurable compression of the catheter segment inside the balloon.

During in vivo evaluation in ten dogs the balloon of the CPC catheter was placed either in the proximal LAD or the proximal LCx. The occlusion tolerance time (OTT), defined as the interval between onset of occlusion and appearance of clearcut signs of ischemia,

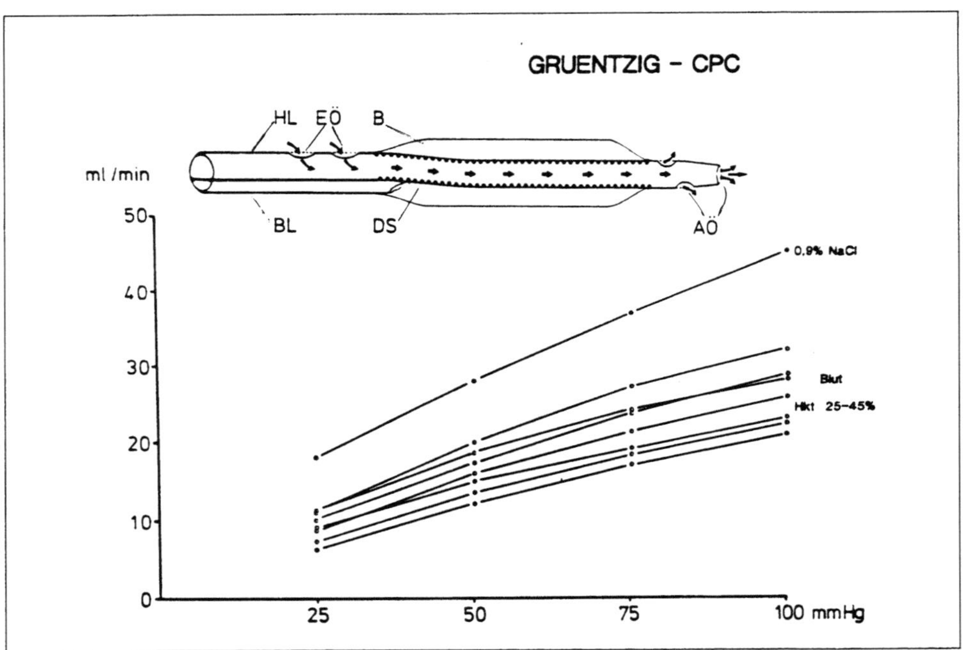

Fig. 3. Pressure/flow relation for the distal segment of the CPC catheter. Insert: Distal part of the catheter; arrows indicate pathway of the blood flow

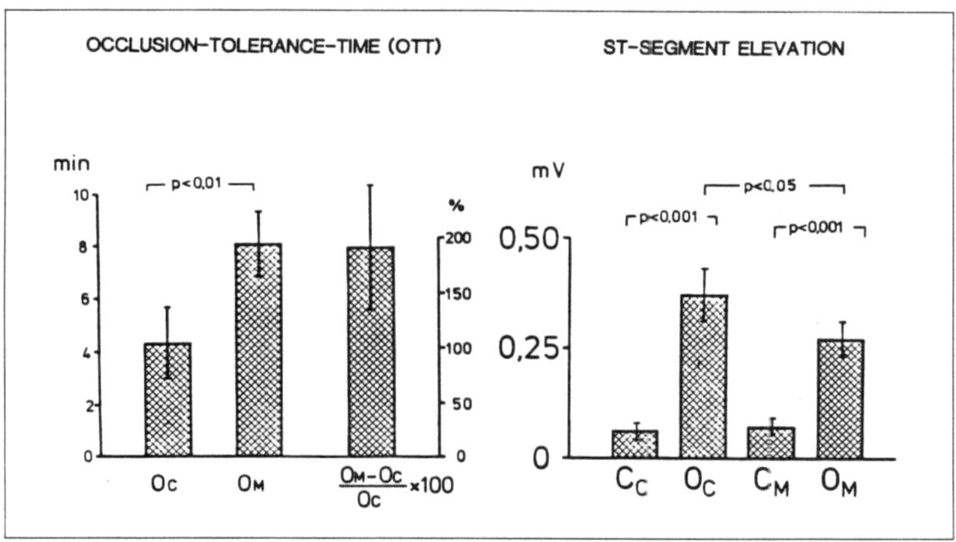

Fig. 4. Occlusion tolerance time and ST-segment shift during conventional occlusion without (Oc) and with continuous perfusion through the CPC catheter (O_M). C_C and C_M are controls prior to balloon occlusion

but with a preset upper limit of 12 min, was then determined. The degree of ST-segment shift in the most sensitive lead was measured as well. Occlusion with passive perfusion (OM) resulted in a significant prolongation of OTT to 486 ± 77 s, whereas it was 256 ± 82 s when blood flow through the distal catheter lumen was blocked during occlusion (OC) ($p < 0.001$, Fig. 4). Subsequent exact ST segment analysis showed less ST elevation at the end of OM (0.22 ± 0.05 mV) than at the end of OC (0.33 ± 0.06 mV, $p < 0.05$). Intracoronary pressure decrease distal to the occlusion was also less with OM than with OC ($P < 0.05$). Hemodynamic data and lactate levels, however, did not show significant differences at the end of OM as compared with OC.

Discussion

Our studies have demonstrated the feasibility of continuous coronary perfusion during PTCA or following PTCA-induced acute coronary occlusion. Both active pump perfusion and the passive form using the CPC catheter clearly had an antiischemic effect. The myocardial protective effect of pump perfusion for a prolonged time period has been shown by others as well [5, 6]. Preliminary results seem to confirm its applicability in man [6]. Our efforts focused on three major problems with active perfusion: a technical one concerning the pump, a hematological one with respect of the degree of induced mechanical hemolysis, and a third dealing with possibilities of adequate pump rate adjustment since, with the current equipment, pressure measurement within the perfused vessel is not possible during perfusion under clinical conditions. Roller pumps used by others have major limitations and, in our opinion, are not suitable, mainly because of very limited pressure output, unreliable flow rate settings – with the flow rate greatly influenced by the pressure output – and unacceptable hemolysis at higher pressures. In comparision, the pump device used by us delivers severalfold higher pump pressures at controllable flow rates, yet with no significant hemolysis even at high pressures. Under certain circumstances, however, still higher pressures than those achieved with the current prototype (15 atm) may be necessary to obtain sufficient flow rates.

The second problem, hemolysis, is determined not only by the pump type, but also by the catheter used for perfusion. Somewhat unexpected was the finding that the difference between catheters in the degree of hemolysis correlates not with the magnitude of flow resistance within the catheter, but rather with the arrangement of the orifices at the catheter tip, i.e., the presence or absence of side holes that cause turbulent, cell-damaging jets.

Our studies have shown that, starting perfusion at a relatively low rate, electrocardiographic monitoring appears to be a sufficiently sensitive guide for flow rate adjustment. Furthermore, there seems to be a rather wide margin of safety, at least in the dog, within which the rate may be varied without greater harm.

Passive coronary perfusion with the CPC catheter, on the other hand, differs from pump perfusion in several respects. First, the highest obtainable flow rates are far below the physiological ones present in major epicardial arteries. Under unfavorable conditions, i.e., with the proximal or distal holes positioned against the vessel wall, flow decreases even further. Second, it depends totally on systemic blood pressure. For both reasons, passive perfusion appears to be least helpful in cases where it would be needed most: in cases with occlusion of a vessel supplying a large area of myocardium, with resultant acute left ventricular failure and shock. Nonetheless, continuous perfusion, even at a greatly reduced rate, most likely has more benefits than only allowing prolongation of balloon inflation times as shown in our animal experiments and also in man [7]. In the absence of shock after acute coronary occlusion the remaining antegrade flow provided by the CPC catheter probably will help to preserve myocardial viability until surgery, not only by a minimum of oxygen supply, but also by washout of accumulating metabolites, with a reduction in local tissue acidosis.

References

1. Grüntzig A (1976) Perkutane Dilatation von Coronarstenosen – Beschreibung eines neuen Kathetersystems. Klin Wochenschr 54: 543–5454
2. Grüntzig A, Riedhammer HH, Turina, M, Rutishauser W (1976) Eine neue Methode zur perkutanen Dilatation von Koronarstenosen – tierexperimentelle Prüfung. Verh Dtsch Ges Kreislaufforsch 42: 282–285
3. Busch U, Erbel R, Clas W, Pfeiffer U, Meyer J, Blümel G, Blömer H (1985) Verbesserte Okklusionstoleranzzeit durch kontinuierliche Koronarperfusion mit einem modifizierten Grüntzig-Koronarangioplastiekatheter. Z Kardiol 74: 435–439
4. Busch U, Pfeiffer U, Babic R, Kursawe U, Sebening H, Blümel G, Blömer H (1986) Selektive Koronardauerperfusion über Angioplastiekatheter nach akutem Gefäßverschluß. Z Kardiol 75: 27–36
5. Meier B, Grüntzig AR, Dekmazian RH, Brown JE (1985) Percutaneous perfusion of occluded coronary arteries with blood from the femoral artery: a dog study. Cathet Cardiovasc Diagn 11: 81–87

6. Hombach V, Höff HW, Fuchs M, Behrenbeck DW, Tauchert M, Hilger HH (1984) Myokardprotektion bei PTCA durch Coronarperfusion mit oxygeniertem Blut. Z Kardiol 73 [Suppl 1]: 61
7. Erbel R, Clas W, Busch UW, von Seelen W, Brennecke R, Blömer H, Meyer J (1985) Modifizierter Ballonkatheter zur kontinuierlichen koronaren Perfusion während perkutaner transluminaler koronarer Angioplastie. Z Kardiol 74 [Suppl 3]: 105

Author's address:
Dr. U. W. Busch
I. Medizinische Klinik
und Poliklinik rechts der Isar
der TU München
Ismaninger Str. 22
8000 München 80

Prevention of Thrombosis in Percutaneous Coronary Angioplasty

M. A. J. Weber, J. Kotzur, A. Zitzmann, M. Haufe, W. Schramm, R. Lorenz, and K. Theisen

Medizinische Klinik Immenstadt, University of Munich

Successful angioplasty includes prevention of thrombosis at the site of dilatation. The pathophysiology of thrombus formation after angioplasty resembles the process at the site of an advanced arteriosclerotic plaque.

Importance of Thrombosis and Antiplatelet Therapy in Coronary Artery Disease

Progression of early lesions in coronary artery disease to hemodynamic relevance is slow. Though platelets are involved in the process, antiplatelet therapy has only recently been shown to be effective [1]. New hope for primary prevention of coronary artery disease has been generated from epidemiologic and experimental studies with dietary eicosapentaenoic acid [2-4].

Progression of the lesion is rapid when thrombus formation occurs at the site of the plaque. This is an important mechanism in unstable angina pectoris and myocardial infarction. Antiplatelet therapy has been effective in these settings. The important questions are why and when does thrombus formation occur at the plaque? An answer was proposed by Virchow as early as 1846. This concept includes a triad of disorders of hemodynamics, hemostasis, and the vessel wall. Following angioplasty, damage to the vessel wall activates the coagulation process and is the main reason for thrombus formation.

Intact endothelial wall prevents thrombus adhesion, e.g., by production of prostacyclin in the endothelial cell. Prostacyclin causes vasodilation and prevents aggregation and thus antagonizes the action of platelet-derived thromboxane, which has the opposite effects. After the vessel wall is damaged due to the angioplasty procedure, platelets adhere to the wall. Platelets are then activated by collagen fibrils and the von Willebrand factor. Subsequently, thromboxane leads to aggregation of further platelets and to vasoconstriction. In addition, platelets also activate intrinsic coagulation through platelet factor 3. In deep lesions, coagulation is also stimulated by tissue thromboplastin and a lack of plasminogen activator and heparin in the vessel wall [1, 5, 6].

The important question of whether there is a general hypercoagulable state in coronary artery disease has not been resolved, but there have been observations that there can be a localized hypercoagulable state if there is a pre-existing thrombus at the lesion which is to be dilated. The thrombus activates platelets by means of thrombin. An occlusion rate of 73% (11/15) after angioplasty in the presence of a thrombus at the dilatation site has been reported, in contrast to only 8% (18/223) in cases without a pre-existing thrombus [7].

Therapeutic Options for Preventing Thrombus Formation in Angioplasty

Acetylsalicylic acid inhibits cyclo-oxygenase and thus both thromboxane and prostacyclin synthesis. The optimal acetylsalicylic acid dosage is not yet established. Low-dose acetylsalicylic acid (100 mg/day) blocks thromboxane [8], yet it decreases prostacyclin production to a lesser degree, thus shifting the balance to the side of antiaggregation. In a randomized trial we showed reduced graft occlusion after coronary bypass surgery with low-dose acetylsalicylic acid [9, 10]. In baboon experiments the drug regimen most effective in preventing thrombus formation in arteriovenous cannulas was high-dose acetylsalicylic acid in combination with dipyridamole [11]. So far, there have been no clinical trials in patients with coronary artery disease comparing different dosages in the same study. The combination with dipyridamole, though promising in animal experiments, has not shown significant additional therapeutic effects in clinical trials [12, 13]. An additional advantage of low-dose acetylsalicylic acid is the low incidence of side effects, and thus improved compliance on the part of patients.

Prevention of Thrombosis Before Angioplasty

There are no reports on how to prevent progression of the lesion or even occlusion during the interval between diagnosis and angioplasty. Nonetheless, preliminary answers can be deduced from data on patients with unstable angina pectoris. The infarction rate in these patients is reported to range from 10% during 12 weeks to 17% during an observation period of 7 days. This emphasizes the considerable risk of progression for patients with unstable angina pectoris who are awaiting angioplasty. Both heparin and acetylsalicylic acid reduced the infarction rates significantly in these trials [14, 15]. For patients with stable angina pectoris, the progression rate is slow and antiplatelet therapy is less important.

Prevention of Thrombosis During Angioplasty

Heparin plays the most important role in the prevention of thrombosis during angioplasty. At the beginning of the procedure a bolus of 10 000 IU is given, followed by a continuous infusion of 2000 IU/h. At the end of the procedure no protamine should be given. Heparin dosage is usually not adjusted, since the conventional partial thromboplastin time measurement takes too long to allow the immediate changes to be monitored. The activated clotting time, used in hemodialysis and cardiopulmonary bypass, supplies immediate information regarding the coagulation situation for subsequent dosage adjustments, because measurements can be made within a few minutes [16].
In addition to heparin, antiplatelet therapy has been instituted. The effect of various platelet-inhibiting drugs on thrombus deposition has been tested in heparinized pigs during angioplasty of the common carotid artery. Of all drugs tested, low-dose acetylsalicylic acid and high doses in combination with dipyridamole showed the best results. Surprisingly, prostacyclin and ticlopidine, known as potent antiplatelet drugs, did not show significant results [17, 18]. Randomized trials with thromboxane receptor blockers have so far not been completed.

Dextran therapy as an adjunct to heparin and acetylsalicylic acid plus dipyridamole during angioplasty did not reduce the acute occlusion rate; it was 10% (10/98) for the dextran group as compared with 9% (7/76) for control patients [19]. We studied the effect of low-dose acetylsalicylic acid (100 mg/day) in addition to heparin and found an acute occlusion rate of 9% (5/54). This rate is comparable to that found with high-dose acetylsalicylic acid, but both dosages have yet to be compared in a controlled trial.

So far, the published data have established the need for antiplatelet therapy during angioplasty. This may result in an increased risk of bleeding in cases of emergency bypass surgery. We measured the surgical blood loss in aortocoronary bypass surgery in 89 patients on low-dose acetylsalicylic acid treatment (100 mg/day) started preoperatively, and compared it with that in a control group of 95 patients. Blood loss was significantly increased in the acetylsalicylic acid group, by about 250 ml. There were no fatal bleeding complications, however, and the reoperation rate was not increased in the acetylsalicylic acid group [20].

Urokinase has been used with success by some groups to decrease thrombus formation around the wire [22]. It should be used if there is a pre-existing thrombus at the lesion.

Prevention of Thrombosis and Restenosis after Angioplasty

A study performed after angioplasty has shown recurrance rates of 27% (34/126) with 325 mg/day acetylcalicylic acid and 36% (44/122) in patients randomized to coumarin [21]. Though the lower recurrence rate for the acetylsalicalic acid fell short of being significant, coumarin at least has no advantage over acetylsalicylic acid in preventing restenosis. The lowest restenosis rate has been reported from centers using high-dose acetylsalicylic acid after angioplasty (1500 mg/day); at this high dose there are certainly antiphlogistic effects in addition to antiplatelet effects [22].

Conclusions

Since many ongoing studies need yet to be evaluated, recommendations have to be preliminary. Acetylsalicylic acid is the drug of choice for prevention of restenosis after PTCA. The low-dose regimen appears to be as effective as high-dose treatment with or without dipyridamole.

In patients with unstable angina pectoris, acetylsalicylic acid should be given immediately to prevent occlusion of high-grade lesions. During angioplasty, heparin in addition to acetylsalicylic acid is an established treatment.

References

1. Fuster, V., Steele, P., Chesebro JH (1985) Role of platelets and thrombosis in coronary atherosclerotic disease and sudden death. J Am Coll Cardiol 5: 175B-184B
2. Siess W, Roth P, Scherer B, Kurzmann J, Boehling B, Weber PC (1980) Platelet-membrane fatty acids, platelet aggregation, and thromboxane formation during a Macherel diet. Lancet 1: 441
3. Lorenz, R, Spengler, U, Fischer, S, Duhm, J, Weber PC (1983) Platelet function, thromboxane formation and blood pressure control during supplementation of the western diet with cod liver oil. Circulation 67: 504-511

4. Kromhout, D., Bosschiefer EB, Lezenne Coulander de C (1985) The inverse relation between fish consumption and 20-year mortality from coronary heart disease. N Engl J Med 312: 1205-1209
5. Eichner ER (1984) Platelets carotids, and coronaries. Am J Med 77: 513-521
6. Baumgartner HR (1984) Blutströmung und Thrombogenese Wechselwirkungen zwischen Blutplättchen, Gerinnungsfaktoren und Gefäßwand. Internist 25: 75-81
7. Mabin TA, Homes DR, Smith HC, Vlietstra RE, Bove AA, Reeder GS, Chesebro JH, Bresnahan JF, Orszulak TA (1985) Intracoronary thrombus: role in coronary occlusion complicating percutaneous transluminal coronary angioplasty. J Am Coll Cardiol 5: 198-202
8. Lorenz R, Siess W, Weber PC (1981) Effects of very low dose versus standard acetylsalicylic acid, dipyridamile and sulfinpyrazone on platelet function and thromboxane formation for man. Eur J Pharmacol 70: 511-518
9. Weber M, von Schacky C, Lorenz R, Meister W, Kotzur J, Reichart B, Theisen K, Weber PC (1984) Niedrig dosierte Acetylsalicylsäure (100 mg/tgl) nach aortokoronarer Bypassoperation. Klin Wochenschr 62: 458–464
10. Lorenz RL, von Schacky C, Weber M, Meister W, Kotzur J, Reichart B, Theisen K, Weber PC (1984) Improved aortocoronary bypass patency by low-dose aspirin (100 mg daily). Effects on platelet aggregation and thromboxane formation. Lancet I: 1261-1264
11. Hanson SR, Harker LA (1985) Effects of platelet-modifying drugs on arterial thromboembolism in baboons. J Clin Invest 75: 1591-1599
12. Brown BG, Aillingham RA, Goede L, Wong M, Fee H, Roth J, Carey J (1981) Improved graft patency with antiplatelet drugs in patients treated for one year following coronary bypass surgery. Am J Cardiol 47: 494 (abstr)
13. The Persantine-Aspirin Reinfarction Study Research Group (1980) Persantine and aspirin in coronary heart disease. Circulation 62: 499–461
14. Telford AM, Wilson C (1981) Trial of heparin versus atenolol in prevention of myocardial infarction. Lancet I: 1225–1228
15. Lewis HD, Davis JW, Archibald DG, Steinke WE, Smitherman TE, Doherty JE, Schnaper HW, LeWinter MM, Linares E, Pouget JM, Sabharwal SC, Chesler E, DeMots H (1983) Protective effects of aspirin against acute myocardial infarction and death in men with unstable angina. N Engl J Med 309: 396-403
16. Preiss DU, Zobeley R (1983) Individuelle Heparin und Protamindosierung in der Herzchirurgie. Klin Wochenschr 61: 1141-1146
17. Chesebro JH, Steele P, Lamb H, Stanson A, Holmes D, Dewanjee M, Badimon L, Fuster V (1984) Balloon angioplasty in pigs: effect of platelet-inhibitor drugs on platelet-thrombus deposition. Eur Heart J 5 [Suppl 1]: 70 (abstr)
18. Steele PM, Chesebro JH, Homes DR, Badimon L, Fuster V (1984) Balloon angioplasty in pigs: comparative effects of platelet-inhibitor drugs. Circulation 70 [Suppl II] 361 (abstr)
19. Swanson KT, Vlietstra RE, Holmes DR, Smith HC, Reeder GS, Bresnahan JF (1984) Efficacy of adjunctive dextran during percutaneous transluminal coronary angioplasty. Am J Cardiol 54: 447-448
20. Weber MAJ, ASAAC Studiengruppe (1985) Aortokoronare Bypassoperation: Vergleich niedrig dosierter Actylsalicylsäure zu Antikoagulation. Z Kardiol 74 [Suppl. 5]: 38 (abstr)
21. Thornton MA, Grüntzig AR, Hollman J, King SB, Douglas JS (1984) Coumadin and aspirin in prevention of recurrence after transluminal coronary angioplasty: a randomized study. Circulation 69: 721-727
22. Kaltenbach M (1984) Neue Technik zur steuerbaren Ballondilatation von Kranzgefäßverengungen. Z Kardiol 73: 669–673

Author's address:
M. A. J. Weber
II. Med. Abteilung
Städt. Krankenhaus München-Neuperlach
Oskar-Maria-Graf-Ring 51
8000 München 83
West Germany

66

Platelets, Prostanoids and Percutaneous Transluminal Coronary Angioplasty

H. Riess

III. Medical Department, Klinikum Großhadern, University of Munich

The high frequency of restenosis is one limitation on the benefit of percutaneous transluminal coronary angioplasty (PTCA). As platelet behaviour is thought to be important in the pathogenesis of vasospasm, early coronary artery occlusion and restenosis, antiplatelet therapy is initiated in most patients undergoing PTCA, despite the fact that clear evidence for the beneficial effect of this therapeutic strategy is still lacking.

II. Angioplasty and platelets

During PTCA the arterial wall will be overstretched, leading to spliting and rupture of the underlying plaque and to tears of the intima (1, 2). Thus, platelets have free access to the exposed subintimal layer; they adhere and undergo activation. During activation, platelets release potent mediators, such as adenosine diphosphate (ADP), arachidonic acid metabolites, hormones and polypeptides. Some of these compounds, especially ADP, thromboxane A_2 (TxA_2) and platelet activating factor attract other circulating platelets to aggregate, thus forming the initial hemostatic plug. In addition, platelet activation is interrelated to the coagulation system. Localized formation of an oversized thrombus, resulting in vaso-occlusion, is normally prevented by counteracting endothelial mediators (3). In addition to thrombus formation at the site of vascular injury, platelets contribute to the migration and proliferation of smooth muscle cells and fibroblasts by the release of platelet-derived growth factor(s) (PDGF) (4). Furthermore, PDGF facilitates the lipid accumulation in smooth muscle cells (5) and shows chemotactic and activating properties for granulocytes and monocytes (6, 7). Thus, platelet activation at the site of PTCA may be important in the pathogenesis of early coronary artery occlusion and restenosis following PTCA. Beyond this, vasoactive mediators released from stimulated platelets (ADP, TxA_2, serotonin) may be responsible for localized vasospasms complicating PTCA.

III. Arachidonic acid metabolism

The current interest focusing on arachidonic acid metabolism (Fig. 1) has increased our understanding of platelet : vessel wall interactions. Briefly, arachidonic acid liberated from the cell membrane is transformed – in addition to other competitive pathways – by

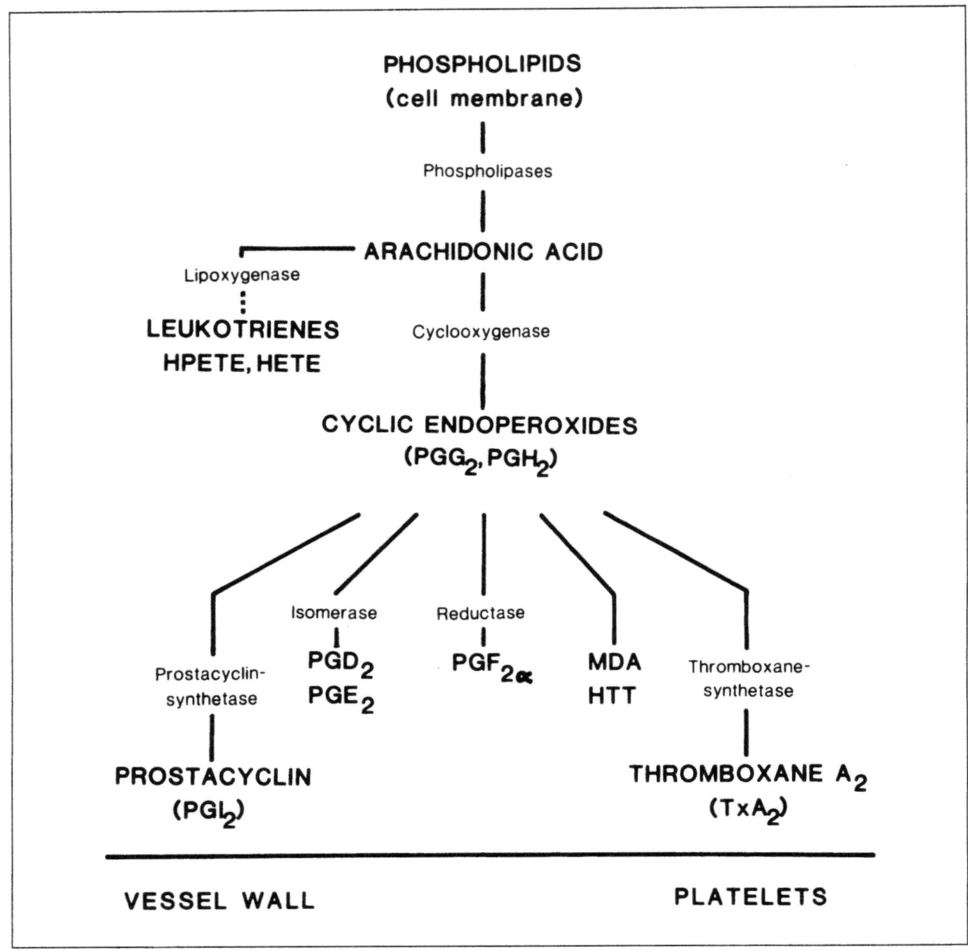

Fig. 1. Arachidonic acid metabolism in platelets and vessel wall (simplified). Abbreviations: HPETE = hydroperoxyeicosateraenoic acid, HEP = hydroxyeicosatetraenoic acid. HTT = hydroxyheptadecatrienoic, MDA = malondialdehyde; PGG_2 = prostaglandin G_2, etc.

cyclooxygenase to cyclic endoperoxides, which in turn are further metabolized to vasoactive prostanoids. Activated platelets mainly generate TxA_2, a potent vasoconstrictor and proaggregatory agent. Its action is balanced by prostacyclin (prostaglandin I_2, PGI_2), a potent vasodilator and antiaggregatory agent, generated mainly by the blood vessel. Currently, these two arachidonic acid metabolites are thought to play a major role in maintaining blood flow.

Several studies have indeed shown a disturbed $TxA_2 : PGI_2$ balance in patients with unstable angina, vasospasm and myocardial infarction as evidenced by: (1) enhanced platelet thromboxane production, (2) decreased prostacyclin production by the arterial wall, (3) decreased platelet-sensitivity to prostacyclin, (4) increased platelet-sensitivity to thromboxane A_2 (8–13).

IV. Antiplatelet medication

When antiplatelet drugs are used in patients, an understanding of the mechanisms of the drug action is necessary. Although some of the drugs commonly used in coronary artery disease, such as nitrates, betablockers, and calcium channel blockers, have weak antiplatelet effects, this is not the rationale for their use in this disease.

The mechanisms responsible for the clinical events of vaso-occlusion, vasospasm and restenosis after PTCA are complex, multifactorial and not completely understood. However, the possibility that platelet-mediated mechanisms play a role in initiating and maintaining these events, forms the basis for the use of antiplatelet drugs. On the basis of the present understanding, it seems reasonable to speculate that the platelet suppressive modulation of arachidonic acid metabolism by drugs, may result in beneficial effects for patients undergoing PTCA. There are several possibilities for altering the arachidonic acid metabolism pharmacologically, some of which are already clinically used whereas others are still under preliminary. We shall describe each in some detail:

Inhibition of phospholipases

Prevention of the release of arachidonic acid from the platelet membrane by blocking phospholipases A_2 and C would abolish thromboxane formation. The agents shown to block arachidonic acid release are corticosteroids, some antimalarial drugs, anesthetics, and phenothiazines.

Corticosteroids act through a soluble protein, synthesized in response to antiinflammatory steroids, thus blocking cyclooxygenase and lipoxygenase pathways (14). However, since platelets cannot synthesize relevant amounts of proteins, TxA_2 production may not be inhibited by corticosteroids. On the other hand, in endothelial cells PGI_2 formation is blocked, because of the synthesis of a protein messenger inhibitor (15). In fact, in a rabbit model hydrocortisone has been found to shorten the bleeding time and to inhibit the production of vascular PGI_2 (16). Thus the overall effect of corticosteroids on the balance between TxA_2 and PGI_2, as well as on platelet aggregation and the prevention of thrombosis, must await further investigation.

Using other phospholipase inhibitors many diverse effects of these agents must be considered. No selective inhibitors of platelet phospholipases have been identified until now.

Inhibition of cyclooxygenase

Aspirin and aspirin-like drugs in vitro and in vivo inhibit platelet aggregation and platelet release reaction, whereas the adhesion of platelets to subendothelium is not affected. In vivo a prolongation of the bleeding time is observed.

Large doses of aspirin (300 to 1500 mg) irreversibly inhibit the cyclooxygenase by acetylation, not only in platelets but also in the vessel wall (17). Thus synthesis of cyclic endoperoxides and TxA_2 as well as of PGI_2 is blocked. Although a light bleeding tendency has been observed in congenital deficiency of TxA_2 and PGI_2 (18), the inhibition of endothelial cyclooxygenase, resulting in decreased PGI_2-synthesis, may be responsible for the unimpressive benefit shown by aspirin in large scale trials with postmyocardial infarction patients (19). On the other hand, two well-designed studies document the life-saving effect of aspirin in unstable angina (20, 21). In contrast to stable angina, there are some similarities between pathophysiological observations made in unstable angina and post-PTCA complications, e.g., rupture of atheroslerotic plaques, formation of platelet thrombi, vasospasm and rapid progression of coronary artery stenosis (22).

Because of the limited protein-synthesizing ability of platelets, the inactivation of the enzyme by a single dose of aspirin will last for the entire platelet life span (about 8 days). On the other hand, cyclooxygenase in the vessel wall is probably less sensitive to aspirin and may be resynthesized. It is on this basis that low or intermittent (twice weekly) doses of aspirin are recommended. This mode of application may preserve cyclooxygenase in the vessel wall due to resynthesis of the enzyme, resulting in a possible shift of the TxA_2 : PGI_2 balance in favour of antithrombogenic effects.

Selective inhibition of platelet cyclooxygenase not only prevents the formation of TxA_2 but also of prothrombogenic cyclic endoperoides (23). In accordance with this hypothesis a hemostasic defect has been reported in platelet cyclooxygenase deficiency (24). At the moment, it remains speculative whether low doses of aspirin can sufficiently alter the balance between TxA_2 and PGI_2 so that thrombus formation can be prevented. The first experimental investigations measuring vessel wall PGI_2 production in the course of low dose aspirin therapy (below 150 mg per day) are contradictory (25, 26). Results of large-scale trials with low dose aspirin are not yet available. The first promising results, in a small group of patients after coronary artery bypass graft surgery, have to be confirmed (27).

The fact that inhibition of platelet cyclooxygenase may shift arachidonic acid metabolism towards the lipoxygenase pathway is of concern. This would result in increased formation of leukotrienes, hydroperoxy- and hydroxy-eicosatetraenoic acids. These highly active metabolites of arachidonic acid may be responsible for aspirin-provoked angina in patients with variant angina (28). Furthermore, these agents may be involved in the stimulation of monocytes and macrophages (29) which by themselves are thought to be important in atherogenesis (30).

Inhibition of thromboxane synthetase

The uncertainty and variability of phospholipase or cyclooxygenase inhibition on the TxA_2: PGI_2 balance, initiated the search for selective inhibitors of thromboxane synthetase, suppressing the production of TxA_2 while sparing that of prostacyclin. However, the use of potent selective thromboxane synthetase inhibitors has raised some doubts about their efficiency as antiaggregating and antithrombotic drugs.

During thromboxane synthetase inhibition, cyclic endoperoxides accumulate and may replace TxA_2 as mediators of platelet activation (31). Furthermore, cyclic endoperoxides will be converted to other prostanoids that may modulate platelet function. PGE_2 and PGD_2, both produced in excess when thromboxane synthetase is blocked, may, respectively, potentiate and inhibit platelet activation by cyclic endoperoxides (32). On the other hand, cyclic endoperoxides released by activated platelets may be utilized by the vessel wall and/or leucocytes, resulting in increased PGI_2 formation (33). The clinical relevance of these phenomena during thromboxane synthetase inhibition is still open to discussion. In man, a slight prolongation of the bleeding time and weak antiaggregatory

70

effects ex vivo have been reported using specific inhibitors of thromboxane synthetase (34). Large clinical studies have begun using this kind of drug. The results will clarify the role of these drugs in conditions where platelet activation is thought to be important.

Antagonists of the thromboxane/endoperoxide receptor

Blockade of the common receptor for thromboxane and cyclic endoperoxides without altering the arachidonic acid metabolism represents an attractive approach to antiplatelet therapy. Several compounds have been characterized as thromboxane receptor antagonists during the last few years. Data from man, however, currently concern mainly BM 13.177, a sulphonamide derivate. Using this reversible and selective thromboxane antagonist in patients with atherosclerotic disease, a significant porlongation of the bleeding time and a time dependent inhibition of platelet aggregation ex vivo was found (35). In addition, plasma levels of β-thromboglobulin and platelet factor 4 decreased during treatment, suggesting reduced intravascular platelet activation (35). In patients undergoing PTCA, we found antiplatelet effects of BM 13.177, comparable to those of aspirin with regard to the prolongation of the bleeding time and ex vivo inhibition of collagen-induced aggregation (36). Follow-up of two groups, each of seven patients, for three months after PTCA revealed no statistically significant difference in restenosis after BM 13.177 as compared with aspirin (36). The results of a placebo-controlled double blind study in patients undergoing PTCA are expected within the next two years. This study and other clinical investigations will help to determine the role of endoperoxides and TxA_2 in PTCA and different clinical conditions. Receptor binding studies using different drugs, as well as investigations into receptor distribution and density are now starting. These data will facilitate the interpretation of clinical results with different drugs in the future.

Stimulation of prostacyclin synthesis

Some drugs used in coronary artery disease and arteriosclerosis obliterans, such as molsidomin and pentoxifyllin are thought to stimulate endothelial PGI_2 synthesis (37, 38). The relevance of this phenomenon, as well as the clinical efficiency of drugs developed in order to stimulate prostacyclin synthetase (39), remains to be established.

Prostacyclin mimetica

The stimulation of adenylate cyclase by PGI_2 increases the intraplasmatic level of cyclic adenosine monophosphate (40). Thus platelet reactivity in response to almost every physiological and pathophysiological stimulus is reduced. In addition to platelet aggregation, platelet adhesion and release reaction are inhibited. The use of PGI_2 as an antithrombotic agent is limited by its short biological half life, the necessity for parenteral application and the vasodilating effects.
More stable PGI_2 analogues which can be applied orally and/or parenterally are under clinical investigation. Up to the present, however, attempts to separate antiplatelet from

vasodilating properties of prostacyclin have not succeeded. Therefore the therapeutic use of these compounds is limited to a few clinical conditions, because of hypotensiv side-effects.

V. Conclusion

The mechanism leading to vasospasm, early coronary artery occlusion and restenosis during and after PTCA are complex, and platelets are involved in various stages. The understanding of platelet: vessel wall as well as platelet : platelet interactions are important in determining the actions of pharmacologic agents. Although it is still uncertain whether alterations in the $TxA_2 : PGI_2$ balance are primary or secondary phenomena in coronary artery disease, it seems likely that modulation of this balance by drugs may have important effects in preventing or limiting the clinical events complicating PTCA. Further clinical investigations will help to establish the optimal therapeutic strategy for patients undergoing PTCA. Specific drugs, working at specific sites, may be more effective than agents used at present. Until definite evidence of inhibition of vasospasm, early coronary artery occlusion and/or restenosis can be demonstrated with the use of platelet-suppressive therapy, only limited recommendations can be made:
Patients undergoing PTCA should be given aspirin with or without dipyridamole. This antiplatelet regime should be started at least one day before PTCA and should be continued for more than three to six months. Derived from the available data, a daily dose of 300 mg of aspirin or more is recommended. In addition to platelet-suppressive therapy, heparin should be given during the procedure of PTCA and for a further 24 hours, in order to prevent early thrombus formation. Drugs such as nitrates, beta blockers, and calcium channel blockers should be continued, if necessary.

References

1. Block PC, Fallon JT, Elmer D (1980) Experimental angioplasty: lessons from the laboratory. AJR 135: 907
2. Block PC, Baughman KL, Pasternak RC, Fallon JT (1980) Transluminal angioplasty: correlation of morphologic and angiographic findings in an experimental model. Circulation 61: 778
3. Gerlach E, Nees S, Becker BF (1985) The vascular endothelium: a survey of some newly evolving biochemical and physiological features. Basic Res Cardiol 80: 457
4. Ross R, Vogel A (1978) The platelet-derived growth factor: a review. Cell 14: 203
5. Witte LD, Cornicelli JA, Miller RW, Goodman DS (1984) Effects of platelet-derived and endothelial cell-derived growth factors on the low density lipoprotein receptor pathway in cultured human fibroblasts. J Biol Chem 257: 5392
6. Denel RF, Senior RM, Huang JS, Griffin GL (1982) Chemotaxic of monocytes and neutrophils to platelet-derived growth factor. J Clin Invest 69: 1046
7. Tzeng DY, Denel RF, Huang JS, Baehner RL (1985) Platelet-derived growth factor promotes human peripheral monocyte activation. Blood 66: 179
8. Lewy RI, Smith JB, Silver JB, Saia J, Walinsky P, Wiener L (1979) Detection of thromboxane B_2 in peripheral blood of patients with Prinzmetals angina. Prostaglandins Med 2: 243

9. Hirsh PD, Hillis LD, Campbell WB, Firth BG, Willerson JT (1981) Release of prostaglandins and thromboxane into the coronary circulation in patients with ischemic heart disease. N Engl J Med 304: 685

10. Fitzgerald GA, Pedersen AK, Patrono C (1983) Analysis of prostacyclin and thromboxane biosynthesis in cardiovascular disease. Circulation 67: 1174

11. Pitt B, Stea MJ, Romson JL, Lucchesi BR (1983) Prostaglandins and prostaglandin inhibitors in ischemic heart disease. Ann Intern Med 99: 83

12. Sinzinger H, Silberbauer K, Geigl W, Wagner O, Winter M, Auerswald W (1979) Prostacyclin activity is diminished in different types of morphologically controlled human atherosclerotic lesions. Thromb. Haemost 42: 803

13. Fitzgerald DJ, Roy L, Catella F, Fitzgerald GA (1986) Platelet activation in unstable coronary disease. N Engl J Med 315: 983

14. Flower RJ, Blackwell GJ (1976) Anti-inflammatory steroids induce biosynthesis of a phospholipase A_2 inhibitor which prevents prostaglandin generation. Nature 278: 456.

15. Jorgensen KA, Stofferson E (1981) Hydrocortisone inhibits platelet prostaglandin and endothelial prostacyclin production. Pharmacol Res Commun 13: 579

16. Blajchman, MA, Senyi AF, Hirsh J (1979) Shortening of the bleeding time in rabbits by hydrocortisone caused inhibition of prostacyclin generation by the vessel wall. J Clin Invest 63: 1026

17. Roth GJ, Siok CJ (1978) Acetylation of the NH_2-terminal serine of prostaglandin synthetase by aspirin. J Biol Chem 253: 3782

18. Parett FI, Mannucci PM, D'Angelo A, Smith JB, Santebin L, Galli G (1980) Congenital deficiency of thromboxane and prostacyclin. Lancet I: 898

19. Bertele V, Salzman, EW (1985) Antithrombotic therapy in coronary artery disease. Artherosclerosis 5: 119

20. Lewis HD, David JW, Archibald DG, Steinke, WE, Smitherman TC, Doherty JE, Schnaper HW, LeWinter MM, Linares E, Pouget JM, Sabharwal SC, Chesler E, DeMots H (1983) Protective effects of aspirin against acute myocardial infarction and death in men with unstable angina. N Engl J Med 309: 396

21. Cairns J, Gent M, Singer J, Finnie K, Froggat G, Holder D, Jablonsky G, Kostuk W, Melendez L, Myers M, Sackett D, Sealey B, Tanser P (1984) A study of aspirin and/or aulfinpyrazone in unstable angina. Circulation 70: 415

22. Fuster, V., Chesebro, JH (1986) Mechanisms of unstable angina N Engl J Med 315: 1023.

23. Rybicki JP, LeBreton GC (1983) Prostaglandin H_2 directly lowers human platelet cAMP levels. Thromb Res 30: 407

24. Malmsten C, Hamberg M, Svensson J, Samuelsson B (1975) Physiological role of an endoperoxide in human platelets: hemostatic defect due to platelet cyclooxygenase deficiency. Proc Natl Acad Sci USA 72: 1446

25. Weksler BB, Pett SB, Alonso D, Richter RC, Stelzer P, Subramanian V, Tack-Goldman K, Gay WA (1983) Differential inhibition by aspirin of vascular and platelet prostaglandin synthesis in atherosclerotic patients. N Engl J Med 308: 800

26. Hanley SP, Bevan J (1985) Inhibition by aspirin of human arterial and venous prostacyclin synthesis. Prostaglandins Leukotrienes Med 20: 141

27. Lorenz RL, Schacky CV, Weber M, Meister W, Kotzur J, Reichardt B, Theisen K, Weber PC (1984) Improved aorto coronary bypass patency by low dose aspirin (100 mg daily). Effect on platelet aggregation and thromboxane formation. Lancet I: 1261

28. Miwa K, Kambara H, Kawai C (1981) Exercise-induced angina provoked by aspirin administration in patients with variant angina. Am J Cardiol 47: 1210

29. Goetzl EJ, Hill HR, Gorman RR (1980) Unique aspects of the modulation of human neutrophils function by 12-hydroperoxy-5,8,10,14-eicosatetraenoic acid. Prostaglandins 19: 71

30. Gerrity RG (1981) Transition of blood borne monocytes into foam cells in fatty lesions. AM J Pathol 103: 181

31. Bertele V, Falanga A, Tomasiak M, Chiabrando C, Cerletti C, de Gaetano G (1984) Pharmacological inhibition of thromboxane synthetase and platelet aggregation: modulatory role of cyclooxygenase products. Blood 63: 1460

32. Heptinstall S, Bevan J, Cockbill SR, Hanley SP, Parry J (1980) Effects of a selective inhibitor of thromboxane synthetase on human blood platelet behaviour. Thromb. Res. 20: 219

33. Schafer AI, Crawford DD, Gibrons MI (1984) Unidirectional transfer of prostaglandin endoperoxides between platelet and endothelial cells. J Clin Invest 73: 1105
34. Vermylen J, Defreyn G, Carreras LO, Machin SJ, Van Schoeren J, Verstraete M (1981) Thromboxane synthetase inhibition as antithrombotic strategy. Lancet I: 1073
35. Riess H, Hiller E, Reinhardt B, Bräuning C (1984) Effects of BM 13.177, a new antiplatelet drug in patients with atherosclerotic disease. Thromb Res 35: 371
36. Riess H, Höfling B, Von Arnim T, Hiller E (1986) Thromboxane receptor blockade versus cyclooxygenase inhibition: antiplatelet effects in patients. Thromb Res 42: 235
37. Sinzinger H (1983) Pentoxifylline enhances formation of prostacyclin from rat vascular and renal tissue. Prostaglandin Leukotrienes Med 12: 217
38. Slany J, Silberbauer K, Sinzinger H, Panzergruber CH (1981) Einfluß von Molsidomin auf die Thrombozytenaggregation und das Prostaglandinsystem. Zschr Kardiol 70: 269
39. Chamone DAF, Vermylen J, Verstraete M (1979) Bay g6575, an antithrombotic compound that stimulates prostacyclin release from the vessel wall. Thromb Haemost 42: 369
40. Moncada S, Vane JR (1979) Arachidonic acid metabolites and the interaction between platelets and blood vessel walls. N Engl J Med 300: 1142

Author's address:
Dr. H. Riess
Medizinische Klinik I
Klinikum Großhadern der Universität München
Marchioninistraße 15
8000 München 70

Coronary Spasm in Patients Treated by Percutaneous Transluminal Coronary Angioplasty

R. Erbel, G. Schreiner, T. Pop, H. J. Rupprecht, and J. Meyer

II. Medical Clinic, Johannes Gutenberg-University, Mainz
Federal Republic of Germany

Summary

The appearance of coronary spasm during PTCA was analyzed in 140 consecutive patients with stable and unstable angina. Coronary spasm was found in 27 patients (19%) and was more common in unstable than in stable angina pectoris (22 versus 5 patients). While coronary spasm could be seen in the first coronary angiogram in 5/27 patients, it developed during the diagnostic procedure in 6/27 patients. In 16/27 patients coronary spasm was induced by the balloon or the guide wire itself.

Twelve of 21 primarily successfully treated patients could be followed up over a 6-month period. Re-stenosis was found in seven patients, two patients suffered myocardial infarctions (3 and 4 months after PTCA), and three patients each had an open vessel.

Cornary spasm is frequently seen in PTCA patients and is more common in unstable than in stable angina pectoris. Coronary spasm during PTCA develops spontaneously or can be induced by the balloon or guide wire. Patients with coronary spasm demonstrated a poor prognosis and a high re-stenosis rate.

Introduction

Percutaneous transluminal coronary angioplasty (PTCA) has become a safe therapeutic procedure in patients with stable angina pectoris [1, 2]. In patients with unstable angina pectoris PTCA can also be performed with a high success rate and low risk [3–5].

Coronary spasm plays a major role in the pathophysiology of unstable angina [6, 7]. Spasm is superimposed on organic lesions as a functional part of the stenosis. In about 90% of patients with coronary spasm, single- or multiple-vessel coronary disease is present [8].

The purpose of this study was to analyze the role of coronary spasm in patients with stable and unstable angina pectoris in whom PTCA was performed.

Methods

The study was performed in 140 consecutive patients. In all patients single-vessel disease was present. We found coronary luminal narrowing of the left anterior descending artery (LAD) in 122 patients, of the right coronary artery (RCA) in 13 patients, and of the left circumflex coronary artery (LCx) in five patients.

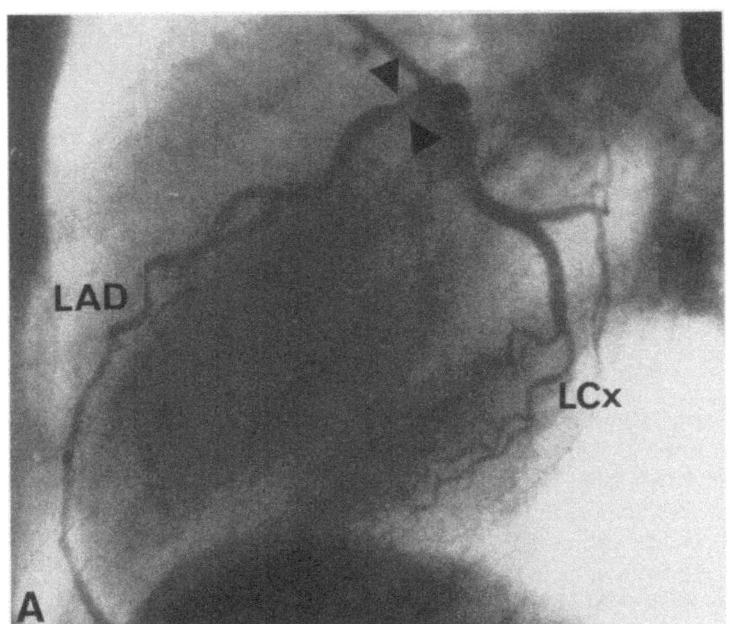

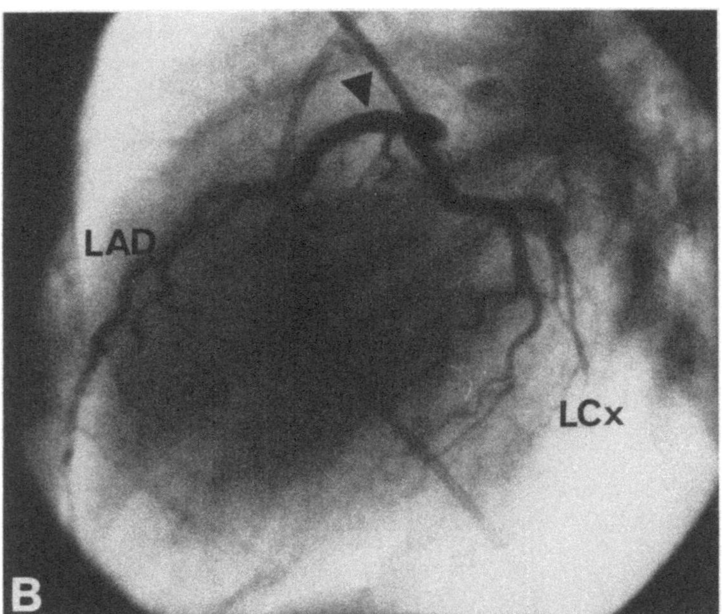

Fig. 1 A, B. Demonstration of coronary spasm (**A**) during the diagnostic procedure and normal coronary vessel at the time of control coronary angiogram (**B**). LAD = Ramus interventricularis anterior, LCx = Ramus circumflexus

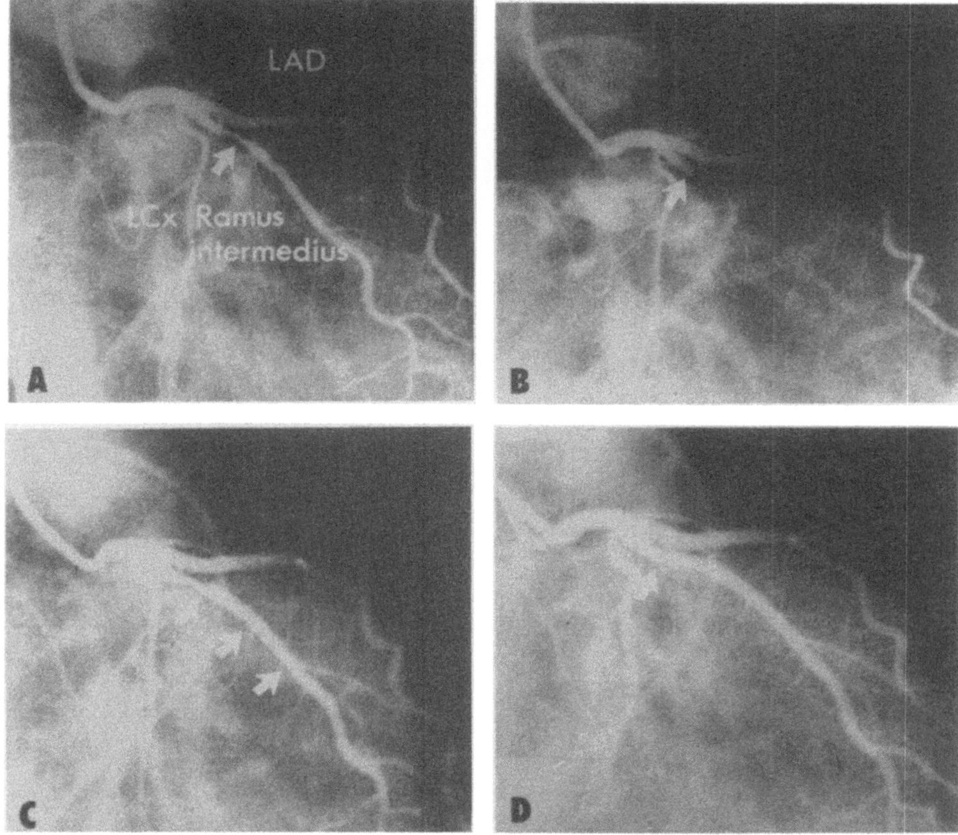

Fig. 2a–d Stenosis of the posterolateral branch of the left circumflex coronary artery (**A**). Spontaneous occlusion with angina pectoris and ST-segment elevation (**B**). Relief after intracoronary injection of nitroglycerine and nifedipine (**C**) and after successful dilatation (**D**). LAD = Ramus interventricularis arterior, LCx = Ramus circumflexus

PTCA was performed as previously described [4]. Patients received 500 mg acetylsalicylic acid and 10 mg nifedipine sublingually the evening before and the morning of the procedure.

In cases of LAD stenosis a Swan-Ganz catheter was positioned within the pulmonary artery, and in cases of RCA stenosis a bipolar catheter with an additional infusion line was advanced into the right ventricle.

Guiding catheters were 9 F. Both steerable and non-steerable Grüntzig balloon catheters were used.

Patients received 10 000 U heparin intravenously prior to balloon insertion. During the procedure dextran (Rheomacrodex) was infused intravenously at a rate of 100 ml/h. After the procedure 0.2 mg nitroglycerine as well as 3000 U heparin were injected intracoronarily. X-ray equipment was a Pandoros U-matic system (Siemens).

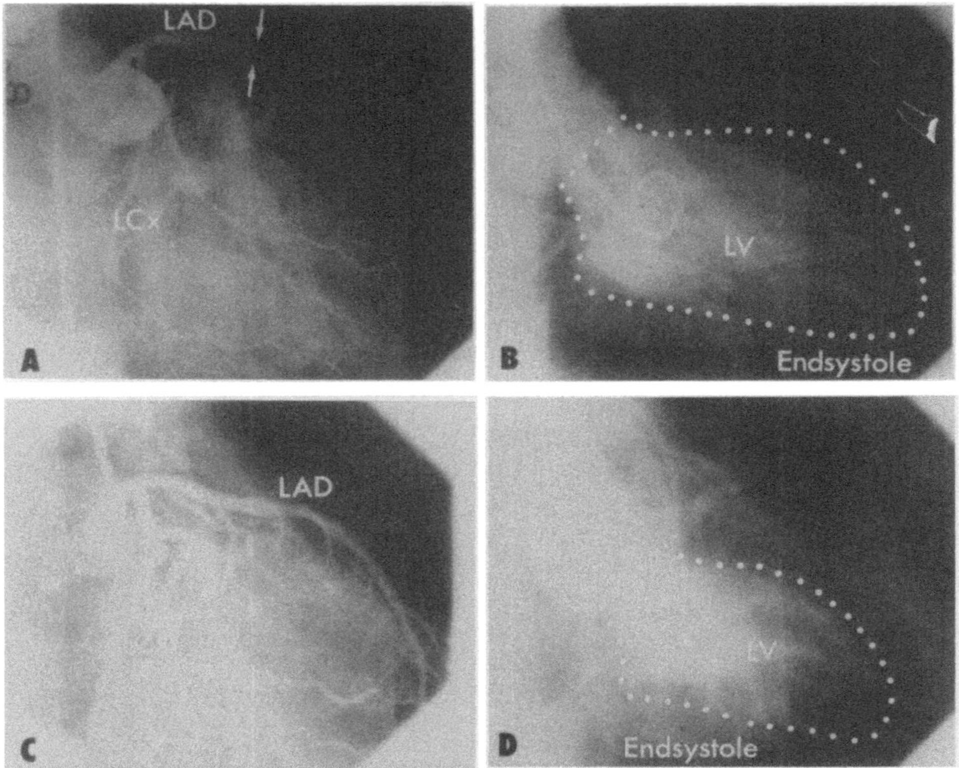

Fig. 3a–d. Total occlusion of the LAD (left arterior descending coronary artery) spontaneously without chest pain **(A)**. End-systolic cineventriculogram of the left ventricle demonstrating enlarged lumen with anterolateral akinesia **(B)**. After relief of the spasm **(C)**, left ventricular function improved significantly **(D)**

Results

In Fig. 1 a coronary angiogram reveals a concentric lesion in the proximal part of the LAD. At the time of the therapeutic procedure, control coronary angiograms demonstrated a normal vessel, suggesting coronary spasm in the first study.

Spontaneous coronary spasm developed in a patient with a stenosis of the posterolateral branch of the LCx. The patient suffered from angina pectoris. ST-segment elevation occurred (Fig. 2). A control coronary angiogram revealed total occlusion of the vessel without any prior manipulation. Injection of nitroglycerine and nifedipine opened the vessel. Successful PTCA was performed.

In a patient transferred to us for PTCA of a proximal LAD lesion a cineventriculogram demonstrated a significantly depressed ventricular function with akinesia of the anterior wall (Fig. 3). Coronary angiography demonstrated a total occlusion of the LAD without angina pectoris, but with slight ST-segment changes. The patient reported only chest discomfort. Additional coronary angiograms after intracoronary injection of nitroglycerine opened the vessel and improved left ventricular function (Fig. 3).

In 27 of the 140 patients (19%) coronary spasm was found, related to the LAD in 22 patients (82%), to the RCA in three (11%), and to the LCx in two (7%). The clinical picture of unstable angina was present in 22 of these 27 patients (80%).

In 5 of the 27 patients (19%) coronary spasm developed spontaneously and was present in the first coronary angiogram. In 6 of the 27 coronary spasm developed during coronary angiography. In 16 of the 27 patients (59%) coronary spasm was induced by the balloon or the guide wire. A typical example is illustrated in Fig. 4. After successful PTCA multiple lesions were apparent in the area of the LCx at the position of the guide wire, resolving after injection of nitroglycerine and nifedipine.

In 99 of the 113 patients (80%) without coronary spasm, PTCA was successful, coronary luminal narrowing was reduced from 73% $\pm$ 12% to 16% $\pm$ 16%. In 21 of the 27 patients (78%) with coronary spasm PTCA was successful; coronary stenoses were reduced from 74% $\pm$ 9.5% to 20% $\pm$ 19%.

Within 6 months' follow-up of 12 of the 21 successfully treated patients, two suffered from myocardial infarctions (3 and 4 months after PTCA), seven developed re-stenoses, and three showed a patent vessel without re-stenosis.

Discussion

PTCA is a successful method of treating patients with stable and unstable angina pectoris [1–5]. Major complications are myocardial infarction due to coronary thrombosis, intimal dissection, and severe spasm [9].

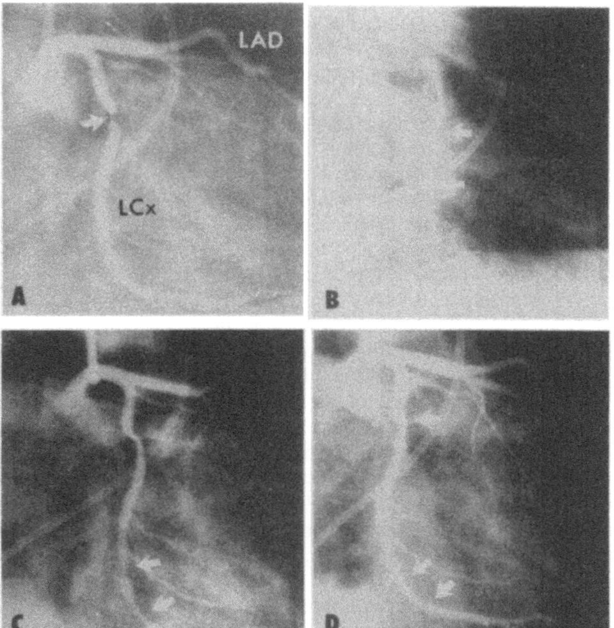

Fig. 4a–d. Coronary stenosis of the left circumflex coronary artery (A). After successful dilatation (B) in the distal part of the vessel, multiple coronary luminal narrowings (C) were seen; these were relieved by nitroglycerine (D)

Coronary spasm in coronary artery disease is found spontaneously in 1%–3% of patients studied in the catheterization laboratory [10]. In patients referred for PTCA, coronary spasm is more common [11, 14]. While 40% of the spasms in our group occurred spontaneously, 60% were induced by the procedure itself, either by the balloon or by the guide wire. Dilatation always stretches the arterial smooth muscle, and this stretching can induce contraction. This mechanism explains why after dilatation pressure increases slowly and shows phasic movement [14]. On the other hand, guide wires can induce spasm by touching the endothelium.

Therapy of patients undergoing PTCA includes nitroglycerine and nifedipine to avoid coronary spasm. In case of coronary spasm an intracoronary injection of both drugs is sometimes needed.

The high re-stenosis rate in our patients, despite a primary success rate nearly egual to that in patients without coronary spasm, could be related in part to unstable angina, as presented in this publication. Patients with unstable angina alone have a higher re-stenosis rate than patients with stable angina [15]. On the other hand, it should be taken into account that the indication for PTCA in patients with coronary spasm can be based only on residual coronary luminal narrowing after maximal vessel dilatation induced by nitroglycerine and nifedipine.

References

1. Grüntzig AR, Senning A, Siegenthaler WE (1979) Nonoperative dilatation of coronary artery stenosis: percutaneous transluminal coronary angioplasty. N Engl J Med 301: 61-68
2. Grüntzig AR (1984) Percutaneous transluminal coronary angioplasty; 6 years' experience. Am Heart J 107: 818-823
3. Meyer J, Böcker B, Erbel R, Bardos P, Messmer BJ, Effert S (1980) Treatment of unstable angina with transluminal coronary angioplasty (PTCA). Circulation 62/III: 160 (abstr)
4. Meyer J, Schmitz H, Erbel R, Kiesslich T, Böcker-Josephs B, Krebs W, Braun PC, Bardos P, Minale C, Messmer BJ, Effert S (1981) Treatment of unstable angina pectoris with percutaneous transluminal coronary angioplasty. Cathet Cardiovasc Diagn 7: 361-371
5. Williams DO, Riley RS, Singh AK, Gewirtz H, Most RS (1981) Evaluation of the role of coronary angioplasty in patients with unstable angina pectoris. Am Heart J 102: 1-9
6. Rafflenbeul W, Smith LR, Rogers WJ, Mantle JA, Racklay CE, Russell RO jr (1979) Quantitative coronary arteriography. Coronary anatomy of patients with unstable angina pectoris reexamined one year after optimal medical therapy. Am J Cardiol 43: 699-707
7. Brown G, Bolson E, Petersen RB, Pierce CD, Dodge (1981) The mechanisms of nitroglycerine actions: stenosis vasodilatation as a major component of the drug response. Circulation 64: 1089-1097
8. Danchin N, Cuilliere M, Cherrier F (1984) Transient acute ischaemic episodes during or immediately after percutaneous transluminal coronary angioplasty. Eur Heart J 5: 362-365
9. Cowley MJ, Dorros G, Kelsey SF, Van Raden M, Detre KM (1984) Acute coronary events associated with percutaneous transluminal coronary angioplasty. Am J Cardiol 53: 12C-16C
10. Lichtlen P (1977) Koronarspasmen während Angiographie. In: P. Lichtlen (ed) Koronarangiographie. perimed, Erlangen, pp 317-324
11. Hollman J, Grüntzig AR, Douglas JS, King SB, Ischinger T, Meier B (1983) Acute occlusion after percutaneous transluminal coronary angioplasty – new approach. Circulation 68: 725-732

12. Erbel R, Meyer J, Effert S (1984) Zum Problem des Koronarspasmus. In: Kardiologie. Grundlagen–Fortschritte–klinische Erfahrungen–Band 1: Die koronare Herzkrankheit. Schattauer, Stuttgart, pp 113-135
13. David PR, Waters DD, Scholl JM, Crepeau J, Sziachcic J, Lesperance J, Hudon G, Bourassa MG (1982) Percutaneous transluminal coronary angioplasty in patients with variant angina. Circulation 66: 695-702
14. Ganz P, Harrington DP, Gaspar J, Barry WH (1983) Phasic pressure gradients across coronary and renal artery stenoses in humans. Am Heart J 106: 1399-1405

Authors' address:
Prof. Dr. med. R. Erbel
II. Medical Clinic
Johannes Gutenberg-University
Langenbeckstr. 1
D-6500 Mainz
Federal Republic of Germany

Incidence of Restenosed Coronary Lesions after PTCA Analysis of Possibly Meaningful Factors

E. Fleck[1], V. Regitz[1], A. Lehnert[1], S. Dacian[2], J. Dirschinger[2], and W. Rudolph[2]

[1] Deutsches Herzzentrum Berlin, Federal Republic of Germany
[2] Deutsches Herzzentrum Munich, Federal Republic of Germany

The attractiveness of balloon dilatation of coronary stenosis as an effective technique for myocardial revascularization is flawed by the failure to achieve a lasting effect in some patients [1, 2]. Published restenosis rates vary between 17% and 40% and appear to depend to a considerable degree on the definition and measurement of restenosis [3–5]. Most studies are based on the visual estimation of the percent of diameter reduction by one or two observers [6]. However, the lack of correlation between the estimated degree of coronary artery stenosis and the measured area reduction has been demonstrated [7, 8]. We therefore designed this study to reliably measure the changes in the angiographically determined stenosis morphology in a large collective and, on the basis of these data, to investigate possible factors favoring restenosis using suitable statistical methods.

Methods

The test series included 110 consecutive patients who had undergone successful coronary angioplasty. In the observation period of 6.6 ± 2 months a total of four patients died: two of sudden death, one of massive cerebral hemorrhage, and one of an acute abdomen. Eleven asymptomatic patients, in whom therefore no high-grade restenosis was suspected, refused follow-up angiography. Thus, the basis for the following analysis is data from angiographic and clinical examination of 95 patients in whom a total of 101 stenoses had been dilated. All of the patients received standard medication with 500 mg acetylsalicylic acid or, if this substance was not tolerated, coumarin (Marcumar), as well as 3 × 20 mg sustained-release nifedipine.

The clinical variables included duration of angina pectoris, age, sex, body weight, blood pressure, presence of diabetes mellitus, and tobacco smoking. Duration of angina pectoris was defined as the time from the onset of symptoms to PTCA. Overweight was diagnosed in accordance with the data of the Metropolitan Life Insurance Company, calculated by means of the body mass index and expressed as percent above the upper limit of normal. Cholesterol, triglyceride, plasma-HDL, and LDL levels, as well as discontinuation of antiplatelet-aggregation therapy were also taken into consideration.

Angiographic variables included the minimum stenotic area in square mm, the percent of area reduction, the presence of a local dissection following PTCA, and the geometry of the stenosis.

The morphology of coronary artery stenosis was quantified with the help of computer-assisted coronary vessel reconstructions, as described earlier [1]. Cross-sectional vessel area was determined proximal and distal to the stenosis and the percent of reduction was derived by comparison with the mean of the proximal and distal vessel areas. Standardization was achieved with the help of the catheter tip. The measurement accuracy was checked by filming catheters and guide wires of various calibers placed in coronary arteries during diagnostic heart catheterization. Using 7-F catheters as a reference, the analysis following the technique described yielded a measurement error of 2.5%–7.7% for diameters of 2.26–0.48 mm, as checked by means of a precision micrometer. The error increased with decreasing diameter.

Based on the potential measurement error, progression of coronary artery stenosis was assumed if the minimum vessel cross section at follow-up had decreased by more than 1 mm^2 in comparison with the acute measurement following PTCA. The collective was divided into three groups: (1) patients with an increase in cross-sectional stenotic area from PTCA to control and patients with a decrease in cross-sectional stenotic area of < 1 mm^2; (2) patients with a reduction of the minimal cross-sectional stenotic area of > 1 mm^2 and a total area reduction of less than 70%; (3) patients with a reduction of the minimal cross-sectional stenotic area of > 1 mm^2 and a total area reduction of more than 70%.

The distribution of the clinical and angiographic variables to the different patient groups was compared using the Student's t-test for quantitative and the chi-square test for qualitative variables. The analysis of possible factors that might influence the restenosis rate was based on a linear multivariance model.

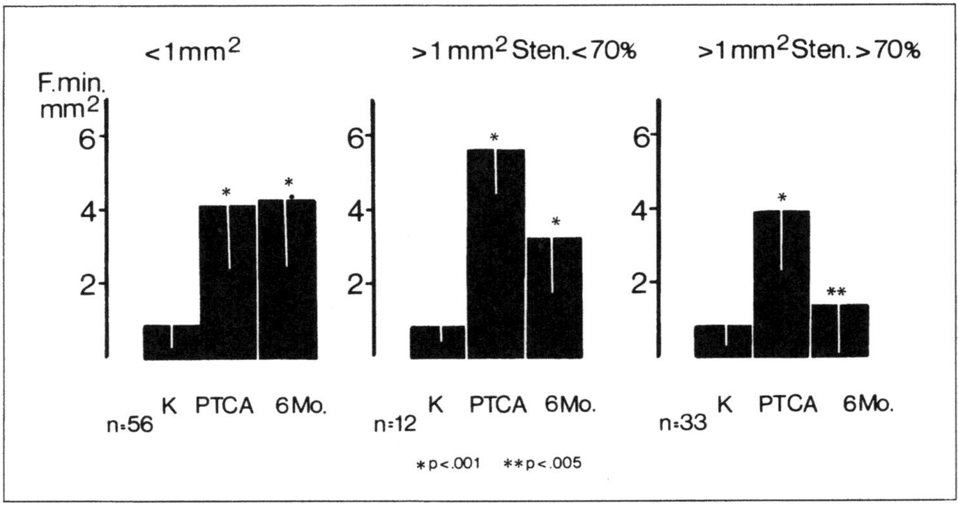

Fig. 1. Minimal cross-sectional area in the region of the stenosis before (C), immediately after (PTCA), and at 6 months post dilatation. < 1 mm^2 = stenosis with change in minimal area (A min) of less than 1 mm^2 or increase in diameter subsequent to PTCA; > 1 mm^2 < 70% = stenosis with reduction in minimal area greater than 1 mm^2 but without rendering luminal narrowing of more than 70%; > 1 mm^2 > 70% = stenosis with reduction in minimal area greater than 70% rendering concomitant luminal narrowing greater than 70%. The three groups were comparable with respect to extent of stenosis prior to PTCA as well as to the increase in minimal area achieved immediately after PTCA. In 45 of the 101 stenoses, however, within the 6-month follow-up period, there was a decrease in minimal area which, in 33 cases, resulted in greater than 70% luminal narrowing

Results

Fifty-six stenoses could be attributed to group 1. The minimal cross-sectional stenotic area before PTCA in this group was 0.83 mm², which was dilated to 4.09 mm² (Fig. 1). After a mean period of 6.8 months following PTCA a mean minimum stenotic area of 4.2 mm² was found. In 17 of these 56 stenoses the measurement after 6.8 months revealed a further increase in the minimum cross-sectional stenotic area as compared with the acute dilatation result.

Twelve stenoses belonged to group 2. Cross-sectional stenotic areas of 0.8 mm² before, 5.5 mm² immediately after, and 3.2 mm² 5.6 months after PTCA were measured in this group. In 33 stenoses in group 3 the corresponding values were 0.8 mm² before, 3.9 mm² immediately after, and 1.4 mm² 6.6 months after dilatation. Altogether, restenosis, i.e., a reduction of more than 1 mm² in the minimum vessel cross-sectional area approximately 6 months after PTCA, was found in 45 of the 101 reangiographed stenoses.

The presentation of the mean values with respect to the percent of area reduction (Fig. 2) yields, in group 1a, mean area reduction from 84% prior to PTCA to 21% immediately after PTCA and 19% half a year later. In group 2, the corresponding mean area reductions were 86% before, 13% immediately after, and 45% about 6 months after dilatation. In group 3, mean area reductions of 85% before, 20% after, and 86% within 6 months were measured.

For multivariate analysis patients were classified into two subgroups with differing severity of progression, i.e., group 1 without significant progression of stenosis and the combined groups 2 and 3 with measurable progression of coronary artery stenosis. No rela-

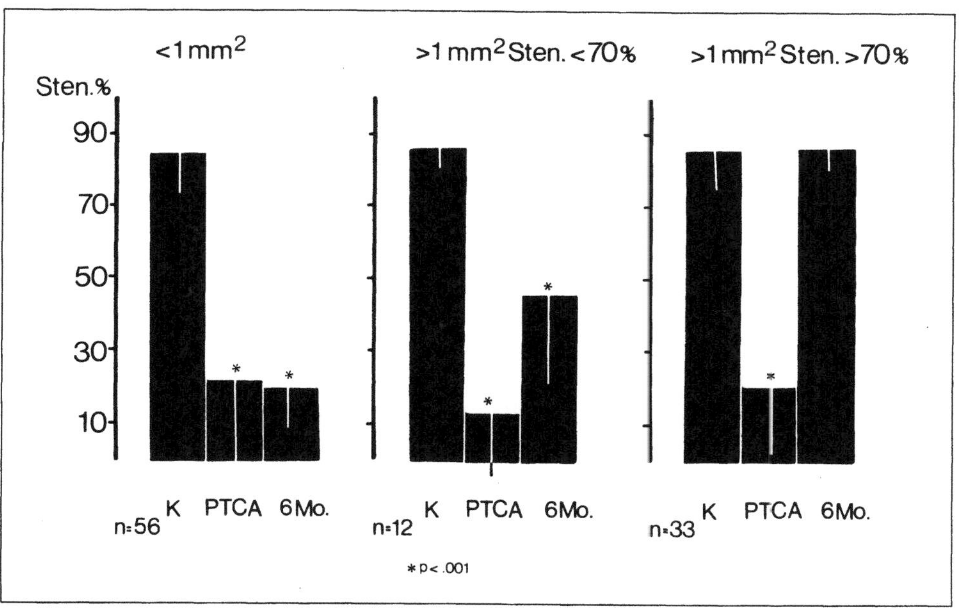

Fig. 2. Minimal area reduction (%) before and after PTCA (for abbreviations and classification see Fig. 1). In 33 of 101 stenoses the extent of narrowing is comparable to that prior to PTCA

Table 1. Analysis of angiographic and clinical data with respect to absence (change in stenosis area < 1 mm²) or presence (change in stenosis area > 1 mm²) of restenosis

Progression	< 1 mm²	> 1 mm²	MV	Student's t-test	CHI²
Stenoses	n = 56	n = 45			
Min. stenotic (mm²) area					
C	0.83 ± 0.57	0.82 ± 0.53		ns	
PTCA	4.05 ± 1.70	4.43 ± 1.64		ns	
6 mo.	4.08 ± 1.66	1.96 ± 1.56		0.001	
Sten. location					
LAD	87%	87%			ns
RCx	11%	4%			ns
RCA	2%	7%			ns
Bypass	–	2%			ns
Sten. form (asym.)	27%	37%	0.411		ns
Local dissection	32%	29%	0.265		ns
Duration of angina pectoris (months)	14.9 ± 38.7	13.8 ± 18.5	0.029	ns	
Age	50.3 ± 8.7	54.3 ± 7.2	0.426	0.01	
Female	14%	7%			ns
Overweight (%)	14.4 ± 9.7	9.6 ± 9.2	0.435	0.01	
Hypertension	58%	42%	0.266		ns
Diabetes	6%	8%			ns
Smoking	55%	44%	0.199		ns
Cholesterol (mmol)	6.23 ± 1.24	5.75 ± 0.91	0.377	0.025	
Triglyc (mmol)	2.15 ± 1.02	1.78 ± 0.89		0.05	
HDL (mmol)	1.18 ± 0.45	1.11 ± 0.34	0.145	ns	
LDL (mmol)	3.98 ± 1.36	3.75 ± 1.06	0.176	ns	
ASA/Warfarin (discont.)	4%	16%	0.451		0.025

MV, Linear multivariance analysis

tionship was found between progression of stenosis and the vessel lumen in the stenotic area immediately after dilatation, the stenosis location, the stenosis morphology, or the angiographic evidence of a local dissection in the dilated area following PTCA (Table 1). There was also no possibility of distinguishing between the two groups by the duration of angina pectoris before PTCA, age, sex, or risk factors such as overweight, arterial hypertension, diabetes mellitus, tobacco consumption, and cholesterol, triglyceride, and HDL and LDL plasma levels. Discontinuation of acetylsalicylic acid therapy, mainly because of gastrointestinal side effects, was more frequently necessary in patients with restenosis.

Discussion

The reported incidence of restenosis after PTCA ranges from 17% to 40% [1, 3, 4, 6]. Visual estimation of coronary artery stenosis may be one of the primary reasons for this variation. The lack of correlation between visual estimation of stenosis and precisely measured stenotic area has been demonstrated in several models [5, 7, 9]. In our study a computer-assisted measuring system was used. The advantages of this system are the great accuracy and reproducibility: both of these qualities have been extensively documented [10–13]. However, infinitely small distances cannot be measured, resulting in a systemic underestimation of high-grade stenoses [1]. This caused no problems in the study presented, as most of the stenoses were distributed in the mean or low range, i.e., stenotic areas of > 1 mm^2.

The search for possible restenosis factors may indicate a weak association between discontinuation of anti-platelet therapy and restenosis. Replacement of acetylsalicylic acid with coumarin, for example in patients with documented ulcus ventriculi after healing of the ulcus, was a possible alternative and is probably not associated with an increased restenosis rate. The missing relationship between most risk factors for arteriosclerosis and restenosis may be explained by the fact that the study interval was too short to document the potential influence of these variables.

One of the interesting findings in this study is that the extent of the intimal lesion and possibly insufficient or excessive dilatation can almost be excluded as restenosis factors, since comparable vessel cross-sectional areas were achieved in all groups after PTCA.

In conclusion, the study demonstrates that within 6 months after PTCA a relatively high incidence of cross-sectional area reductions must be expected. Taking into account our 11 patients who were not reangiographed and in whom no anamnestic evidence of an effective coronary artery stenosis was present, we calculated a restenosis rate of 29%. This is comparable to those in other studies [14–16]. Special attention should be paid to the small group of patients in whom no high-grade stenoses or no angina pectoris reappeared, although a progression has to be assumed based on a reduction of the cross-sectional vessel area in the first 6 months after PTCA. At present, the development of these medium-grade restenoses cannot be predicted.

If they are added to the high-grade restenoses, the total stenosis rate amounts to roughly 40%. Comparable results have been obtained in studies in which dilated coronary artery segments were quantitated using a videodensitometric procedure [1, 5]. This potential incidence of restenosis may be particularly important if multiple dilatations in multiple-vessel disease are considered.

References

1. Fleck E, Dirschinger J, Rudolph W (1985) Quantitative Koronarangiographie vor und nach PTCA. Restenosierungsrate, Analyse beeinflussender Faktoren. Herz 10: 313
2. Grüntzig AR, Sennig A, Siegenthaler WE (1979) Nonoperative dilatation of coronary artery stenosis. N Engl J Med 301: 61
3. Kent KM, Bentivoglio LG, Block PV, Bourassa MG, Cowley MJ, Dorros G, Detre KM, Gosselin AJ, Grüntzig AR, Kelsey SF, Mock MB, Mullin SM, Passamani ER, Myler RK, Simpson J, Stertzer SH, von Raden MJ, Williams DO (1984) Long-term efficacy of PTCA: report of the NHLBI-PTCA registry. Am J Cardiol 53: 27C
4. Levine S, Ewels CJ, Rosing DR, Kent KM (1985) Coronary angioplasty: clinical and angiographic follow-up. Am J Cardiol 55: 673
5. Serruys PW, Reiber JHC, Wijus W, vd Brand M, Kooijman CJ, ten Katen HJ, Hugenholtz PG (1984) Assessment of PTCA by quantitative coronary angiography: diameter versus densitometric area measurements. Am J Cardiol 54: 482

6. Kaltenbach M, Kober G, Scherer D, Vallbracht C (1985) Recurrence rate after successful coronary angioplasty. Eur Heart J 6: 276
7. Harrison DG, White CW, Hiratzka LF, Boty DB, Barnes DH, Eastham CL, Marcus ML (1984) The value of lesion cross-sectional area determined by quantitative coronary angiography in assessing the physiologic significance of proximal left anterior descending coronary arterial stenoses. Circulation 69: 1111
8. White CW, Wright CB, Doty DB, Kiratza LF, Eastham CL, Harrison DG, Marcus ML (1984) Does visual interpretation of the coronary arteriogram predict the physiologic importance of a coronary stenosis? N Engl J Med 310: 819
9. Scoblionko DP, Brown BG, Mitten S, Caldwell JH, Kennedy JW, Bolson EL, Dodge HT (1984) A new digital electronic caliper for measurement of coronary arterial stenosis: comparison with visual estimates and computer-assisted measurements. Am J Cardiol 53: 689
10. Gottwik MG, Siebes M, Kirkeeide R, Schaper W (1984) Haemodynamik von Koronarstenosen. Z Kardiol [Suppl 2]: 47
11. Siebes M (1981) Quantitative Angiographie. Diplomarbeit, Gießen
12. Siebes, M, Kirkeeide R, Gottwik M, Stammler G, Winkler B, Schaper W (1981) Computergestützte Geometriebestimmung und Berechnung der Druckfallfluß-Verhältnisse von angiographisch dargestellten Modellstenosen. Biomed Tech (Berlin) 26: 66
13. Kirkeeide RL, Wüsten B, Gottwik M (1981) Computer-assisted evaluation of angiographic findings. In: Breddin U (ed) Atherogenese. Pathophysiologie und Therapie der arteriellen Verschlußkrankheit. Witzstrock, Baden-Baden, pp 414–417
14. Bentivoglio LG, van Raden MJ, Kelsey SF, Detre KM (1984) PTCA in patients with relative contraindications: results of the NHLBI-PTCA registry. Am J Cardiol 53: 82 C
15. Detre KM, Myler RK, Kelsey SF, van Raden M, Mitchell TH (1984) Baseline characteristics of patients in the NHLBI-PTCA registry. Proceedings of the NHLBI on the outcome of PTCA. Am J Cardiol 53: 7 C
16. Holmes DR, Vlietstra RE, Smitz HL, Vetrovec GW, Kent KM, Cowley MJ, Faxon DP, Grüntzig AR, Kelsey SF, Detre KM, van Raden MJ, Mock MB (1984) Restenosis after PTCA: a report from the PTCA registry of NHLBI. Am J Cardiol 53: 77 C

Authors' address:
Prof. Dr. E. Fleck
Deutsches Herzzentrum Berlin
Augustenburger Platz 1
1000 Berlin 65

Influence of Balloon Size on Recurrence Rate of Coronary Artery Stenosis. Results of a Prospective Investigation

R. von Essen, R. Uebis, B. Bertram, H. J. Schmitz, K. Seiger, and S. Effert

Abteilung Innere Medizin I der Rheinisch-Westfälisch Technische Hochschule Aachen, Federal Republic of Germany

Restenosis of a successfully dilated coronary artery is one of the problems of coronary angioplasty. There are three definitions of restenosis: (a) loss of initial gain of the diameter of more than 20%, (b) loss of more than 50% of initial gain, and (c) restenosis of more than 30% of initial gain. As the definition for a successful angioplasty is an increase of the diameter of the dilated vessel of more than 20%, the first defintion of a restenosis seems to be the most reasonable one. However, different groups use differen: definitions when reporting restenosis rates. Therefore, it is difficult to compare long-term results with regard to the recurrence rates of different centers; they range from 12% to 36% [1–5, 11]. Restenosis may be influenced by selection of patients, technique used for dilatation, medical treatment before, during, and after PTCA, and treatment and elimination of risk factors (see Table 1).

In a retrospective study we demonstrated that the degree of the residual stenosis after successful PTCA influenced the recurrence rate. In 20 patients with restenosis the diameter of the stenotic area after PTCA was significantly lower compared with a group of patients with good long-term results (2.3 ± 0.4 mm versus 2.7 ± 0.5 mm, $P < 0.005$) [6]. However, in this study only patients with concentric stenosis were investigated and these good long-term results were mainly achieved by using larger balloons. Angioplasty is known to produce its effect primarily through mechanical deformation of the arterial wall. Signif-

Table 1. Factors that may influence the restenosis rate

● Selection of patients	− stable or unstable angina − eccentric or concentric stenosis − long or short stenosis
● Technique used for dilatation	− duration of inflation − number of inflations − pressure used for inflation − size of balloon compared with vessel
● Medical treatment	− before, during, and after PTCA − nitrates − calcium channel blockers − anticoagulants
● Risk factors	− smoking after PTCA − cholesterol level (LDL, VLDL)

icant changes are produced, including intimal splitting, intimal-medial dehiscence, and medial necrosis. Repair of the vessel is generally complete, with enlargement of the vessel lumen due in part to permanent stretching of the arterial media [7]. In a second prospective study we therefore (a) investigated the risk of using large balloons without changing the medication before, during, and after PTCA (Table 2) and (b) determined the recurrence rate 6 months after the procedure by a control angiogram.

Table 2. Medication before, during, and after PTCA

Before	acetylsalicylic acid	500 mg p.o.
	nifedipine	10 mg p.o.
During	heparin	10 000 U i.v.
	nitroglycerine	0.2 mg i.c.
After	acetylsalicylic acid	1 × 500 mg p.o.
	nifedipine (at least 6 months)	3 × 10 mg p.o.

Patients and Methods

In a consecutive series of 107 PTCA procedures we were able to pass the stenotic area with the balloon in 100 cases. Fifty-eight patients had an LAD, 26 an RCA, and 16 an RCX stenosis. Sixty-five were concentric and 35 eccentric. We measured the vessel on both sides of the stenosis after i.c. injection of 0.2 mg nitroglycerine in two right-angled projections on a frozen frame. For calibration we used the tip of the guiding catheter (9F = 3 mm). If the diameter of the vessel to be dilated was smaller than 3.4 mm, we used a 3.7 balloon (only Schneider-Grüntzig catheters were used). The balloon size was measured before introduction into the vessel with a pressure of 7 atm and after the procedure with the same pressure as that used during PTCA. Time of inflation was 40 s. The inflation pressure depended on a diagram that correlates increased pressure with the size of the balloon. A remaining pressure gradient of less than 16 mm Hg and a control angiogram performed immediately after PTCA were used to assess primary success. Two right-angled projections with the inflated balloon in the stenotic area were used to correlate the balloon size with the diameter of the vessel.

Results

In all 100 patients in whom we could pass the stenotic area with the balloon, an increase in the diameter of more than 20% was achieved. Comparison with the coronary artery on both sides of the stenosis, the inflated balloon during the PTCA procedure (measured on the cine film) was 1.1 ± 0.14 SD times larger. Mean diameter stenosis before PTCA was 72.3% ± 9.9% (± SD) (= 0.82 ± 0.33 mm) and after PTCA 27.1% ± 12.1% (= 2.18 ± 0.47 mm) (see Fig. 1).

90

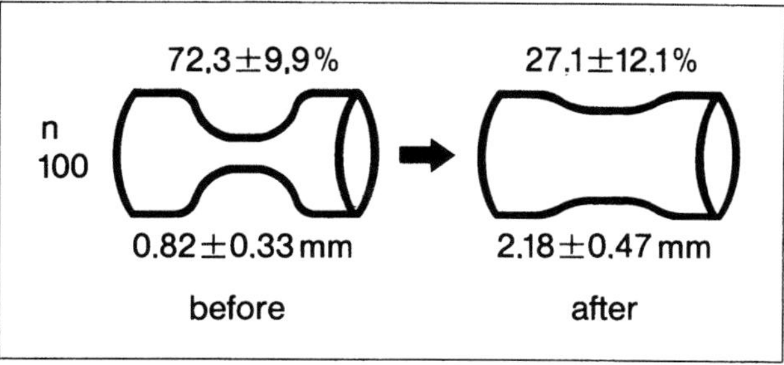

Fig. 1. Stenosis before and after PTCA in 100 procedures

In 47 patients no lesions could be seen in the dilated area. In 42 patients a small wall lesion with a spot of contrast medium in the region of the balloon was observed. Eleven patients developed a dissection which extended the length of the balloon. Three of the latter underwent emergency bypass surgery (3%). Two had an LAD and one an RCA stenosis.

A control angiogram was performed in 89 of these 100 patients 5.9 ± 2.1 months after the PTCA procedure. The three patients who had undergone bypass surgery had no control performed and eight patients refused a second angiogram because they were free of symptoms.

Recurrence Rate

Restenosis was found according to definition 1 (loss of initial gain of more than 20%) in 17 patients (= 19.1%), according to definition 2 (loss of more than 50% of initial gain) in 22 patients (= 24.7%), and according to definition 3 (re-stenosis of more than 30% of initial gain, NHLBI) in 23 patients (25.8%).

The restenosis rate was higher in patients with eccentric stenosis (10/32 = 31.3%, def. 3) than in patients with concentric stenosis (13/57 = 22.8%). In both groups (concentric and eccentric) dissection of the dilated vessel without emergency bypass surgery had a high recurrence rate. However, patients with a wall lesion in the stenotic area after PTCA had the lowest restenosis rate (def. 3; see Fig. 2) if the stenosis was concentric.

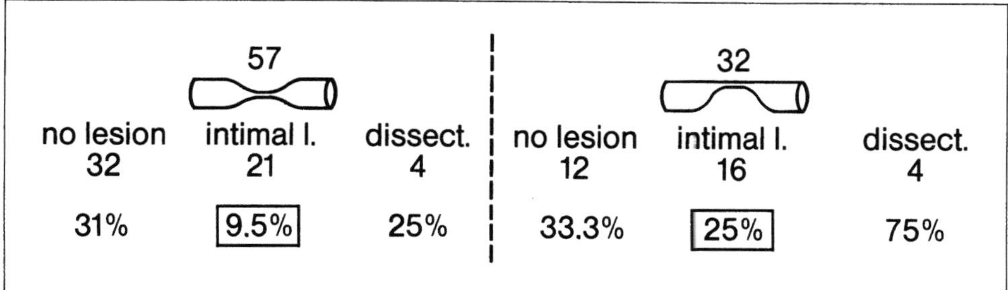

Fig. 2. Restenosis rate according to concentric and eccentric stenosis

Discussion

To date, the manner of determining a restenosis after PTCA is unsatisfactory, as it is dependent on the diameter stenosis in percent before PTCA and not on the absolute diameter of the stenotic area measured in mm². The diameter of the stenosis in percent, however, depends on the diameter of the coronary artery on both sides of the stenosis and is therefore influenced by the tone of the vessel. After vasodilatation due to nitroglycerine or nifedipine the stenosis is calculated to be higher if these drugs increase the diameter of the artery on both sides of the stenosis but not the stenosis area itself. This is the case with most concentric stenoses. One aim of this study was to investigate whether the use of large balloons does bear a higher risk of extensive dissections and emergency bypass surgery. Although the number of patients who underwent bypass surgery was small (3%), and low in comparison with other groups [2, 8–10], the incidence of dissections was relatively high (11%). Four of these patients had an eccentric stenosis of the proximal part of the right coronary artery located in a bend. Therefore, with this type of stenosis one should be cautious in using large balloons.

With regard to recurrence, our results are somewhat disappointing; although the overall rate between 19.1% and 25.8% (depending on the definition used) is lower than that published by the National Heart, Lung, and Blood Institute (33.6%) [11], it is still higher than that published by the Frankfurt group [1].

One explanation might be that 30% of our patients had an unstable angina with an increase in symptoms during the last few weeks before PTCA (some had to be treated with intravenous nitroglycerine and calcium channel blockers). The recurrence rate was higher in these patients than in patients with stable angina [12]. Another explanation may be that restenosis is influenced not only by the mechanical stretching of the wall but also by physiological factors which accelerate the atherosclerotic process (thromboxane A2 and platelet-derived growth factor) [12] and which are not influenced by the size of the balloon but might be influenced by the medication during and after PTCA.

An interesting aspect of our results is the different recurrence rates for eccentric and concentric stenoses: If a small wall lesion is visible the restenosis rate seems to be lower in patients with concentric stenosis (9.5% vs. 25%). However, statistically, this difference is not significant. A visible lesion in the stenotic area after PTCA probably means a small tear in the intima and media and indicates a damaged wall. This coincides with a low recurrence rate, especially in patients with concentric stenosis.

In conclusion, the use of large balloons adequate to the dilated vessel bears a higher risk of dissection, especially in eccentric proximal RCA stenosis. The reduction of the recurrence rate overall is disappointing. However, in concentric stenosis with a small wall lesion after PTCA, the recurrence rate is less than 10%.

References

1. Kaltenbach M (1984) Rezidivhäufigkeit nach erfolgreicher Ballondilatation von Kranzarterienstenosen. Z Kardiol 73 [Suppl 2]: 161–166
2. Kent KM, Bonow RO, Rosing DR, Ewels CJ, Lipson LC, McIntosh CL, Bacharach S, Green M, Epstein SE (1982) Improved myocardial function during exercise after successful percutaneous transluminal coronary angioplasty. N Engl J Med 306: 441–446

3. Meier B, Grüntzig AR, Siegenthaler WE, Schlumpf M (1983) Long-term exercise performance after percutaneous transluminal coronary angioplasty and coronary artery bypass grafting. Circulation 68: 796–802
4. Thornton MA, Grüntzig AR, Hollman J, King SB, Douglas JS (1984) Coumadin and aspirin in prevention of recurrence after transluminal coronary angioplasty: a randomized study. Circulation 69: 721–727
5. Scholl JM, Chaitman BR, David PR, Dupras G, Brévers G, Guiteras Val P, Crepéau J, Lespérance J, Bourassa MG (1982) Exercise electrocardiography and myocardial scintigraphy in the serial evaluation of the results of percutaneous transluminal coronary angioplasty. Circulation 66 (2): 380–390
6. Schmitz HJ, von Essen R, Meyer J,Effert S (1984) The role of balloon size for acute and late angiographic results in coronary angioplasty. Circulation 70 [Suppl II]: 295
7. Castaneda-Zuniga W (1984) Pathophysiologiy of transluminal angioplasty. Improvement of myocardial perfusion. September, Mainz (abstr 15)
8. Dorros G, Cowley MJ, Simpson J, Bentivoglio LG, Block PC, Bourassa M, Detre K, Gosselin AJ, Grüntzig AR, Kelsey SF, Kent KM, Mock MB, Mullin SM, Myler RK, Passamani ER, Stertzer SH, Williams DO (1983) Percutaneous transluminal coronary angioplasty: report of complications from the National Heart, Lung and Blood Institute PTCA Registry. Circulation 67: 723–730
9. Marco J (1983) Angioplastie transluminale des artères coronaires. Arch Mal Coeur 76: 363–369
10. Kent KM, Bentivoglio LG, Block PC, Cowley MJ, Dorros G, Gosselin AJ, Grüntzig A, Myler RK, Simpson J, Stertzer SH, Williams DO, Fisher L, Gillespie MJ, Detre K, Kelsey S, Mullin SM, Mock MB (1982) Percutaneous transluminal coronary angioplasty: report from the Registry of the national Heart, Lung, and Blood Institute. Am J Cardiol 49: 2011–2020
11. Holmes D, Vlietstra R, Smith H, Kent K, Bentivoglio L, Block P, Dorros G, Gosselin A, Grüntzig A, Myler R, Simpson J, Sterzer S, Williams D, Bourassa M, Vetrovec G, Kelsey S, Detre K, Passamani E, van Raden M, Mock M (1983) Restenosis following percutaneous transluminal coronary angioplasty (PICA) – a report from the NHLBI registry. Circulation [Suppl III] 95
12. David PR, Water DD, Scholl JM, Crepéau J, Szlachcic J, Lesperance J, Hudon G, Bourassa MG (1982) Percutaneous transluminal coronary angioplasty in patients with variant angina. Circulation 66: 695
13. Block PC (1984) Arterial reaction to angioplasty: does angioplasty accelerate or improve atherosclerosis? Improvement of myocardial perfusion, September, Mainz (abstr 16)

Authors' address:
Prof. Dr. R. von Essen
Stiftsklinikum Augustinum
Medizinische Klinik B
Wolkerweg 16
8000 München 70

Significance of the Angiographic Coronary Morphology for the Early Outcome of PTCA

T. Ischinger

Division of Cardiology, Klinikum München-Bogenhausen,
Federal Republic of Germany

One limitation of coronary angioplasty is the poor predictability of the reaction of the stenoses to mechanical dilatation. The most frequent coronary vascular complications associated with coronary angioplasty are obstructive coronary dissection or total coronary occlusion, which may lead to acute myocardial ischemia. In about 5% of patients treated with coronary angioplasty, urgent coronary bypass operations are performed in order to minimize the ischemic insult to the myocardium. However, even though expertise and catheter technology of coronary angioplasty have markedly improved, myocardial infarction is still a complication of PTCA, occurring at a rate of 3% in the overall experience.

Therefore, efforts have been made to identify angiographic factors that may predict the outcome and the risk of complications of PTCA [1, 2].

In general, when coronary arteriograms are evaluated in the selection of patients for coronary angioplasty, the following issues are addressed:

1. Feasibility of PTCA
2. Safety of PTCA
3. PTCA strategy
4. Chance of success of PTCA in comparison with the potential of coronary artery bypass surgery

The overriding issue, certainly, is the safety of the procedure for the patient, which depends on the estimated risk of coronary vascular complications and on the expected hemodynamic (clinical) consequence an iatrogenic total coronary occlusion would have for the patient. The immediate clinical risk of PTCA is proprionate to the amount of myocardium which is in jeopardy in the event of ischemic complication. Dilatation of proximal stenoses in vessels with great functional significance e.g., with a large distribution, particularly with a large poststenotic supply area, is associated with an increased clinical risk. It is estimated that if more than 50% of the left ventricular myocardium is rendered acutely ischemic, critical impairment of left ventricular pump function will occur, so that the patient's circulation cannot be sustained through immediate coronary bypass surgery. For this reason, a left main stenosis is considered a relative contraindication. A similar risk may be associated with PTCA in the presence of a totally occluded coronary artery outside of the distribution of the PTCA vessel. Also in patients with previous myocardial infarctions the combination of the previous and the acute ischemic insult may lead to extensive left ventricular damage. Therefore, estimation of the residual amount of viable myocardium that would be left in case of acute occlusion of the PTCA vessel is essential for the assessment of the risk of PTCA in these patients.

The presence of coronary collaterals may markedly modify the risk of a PTCA procedure; if coronary collaterals that supply viable myocardium are originating from the PTCA vessel the mass of myocardium in jeopardy will increase. If the target vessel is receiving angiographically visible coronary collaterals, myocardial ischemia may not occur or may be less severe in case of acute cessation of antegrade flow in the PTCA vessel. While the extent of myocardial ischemia resulting from an acute coronary obstruction may usually be predicted from the diagnosic arteriogram, the occurrence of the coronary vascular complication itself, such as coronary dissection or total occlusion, appears to be less forseeable. However, recent studies have been successful in identifying some angiographic "risk factors" for such coronary vascular complications [2, 3, 6, 9].
The importance of the site of the coronary lesion has been emphasized by several studies. Lower success rates and a higher rate of emergency coronary surgery have been reported with PTCA attempts in the right coronary artery than with those in the left anterior descending and left circumflex arteries [3]. This may be due partially to the tortuosity of the right coronary artery, which may present technical difficulties with advancement of the dilatation system and an increased risk of dissection due to balloon inflation in a bend of the coronary artery.

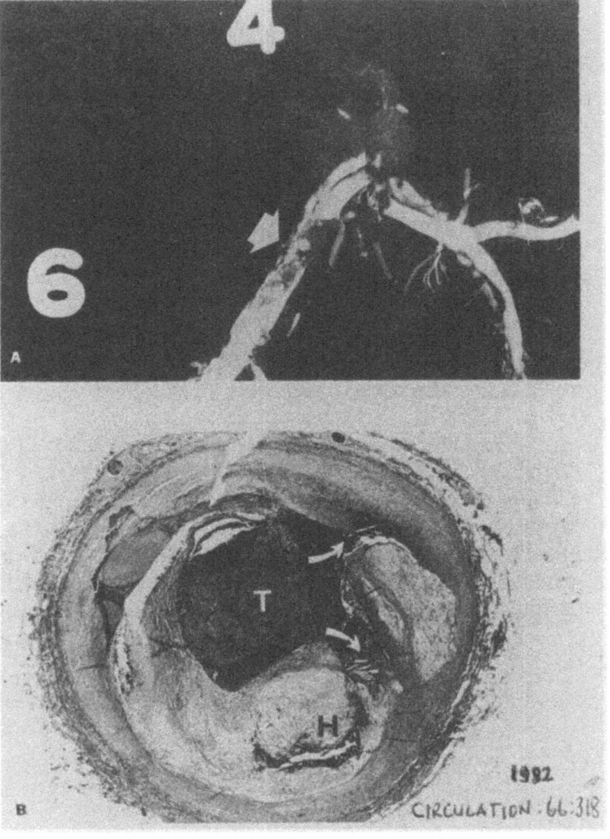

Fig. 1. A Postmortem angiogram of a complicated lesion (LAD, arrow). The borders of the lesion are irregular and there are intraluminal lucencies (filling defects) within the stenosis. B The histologic section shows a "complicated" atherosclerotic plaque with plaque rupture (arrows), intraplaque hemorrhage (H) and intraluminal thrombus (T). (From reference 4 with permission from Circulation)

Angiographic properties of the stenosis itself may also influence the outcome of PTCA. Usually, the analysis of coronary arteriograms describes the obstructive coronary disease in terms of localization and degree of the coronary lesions. Other characteristics of the angiographic morphology of the coronary stenosis have attracted less attention and have not been considered in the routine interpretation of coronary angiograms.

Atherosclerotic coronary obstruction is a complex process leading to fatty, fibrous, or "complicated" plaques [4]. Complicated lesions may be associated with plaque-rupture, ulceration, subintimal hemorrhage or superimposed or recanalized thrombus. These histopathologic properties of complicated atherosclerotic plaques correspond to certain typical angiographic characteristics, as the correlation of pathohistologic and angiographic postmortem studies have shown (Fig. 1) [4]. Angiographically, complicated stenosis morphology is defined as marked irregularity of the stenosis border and/or intraluminal lucency (Figs. 2–4).

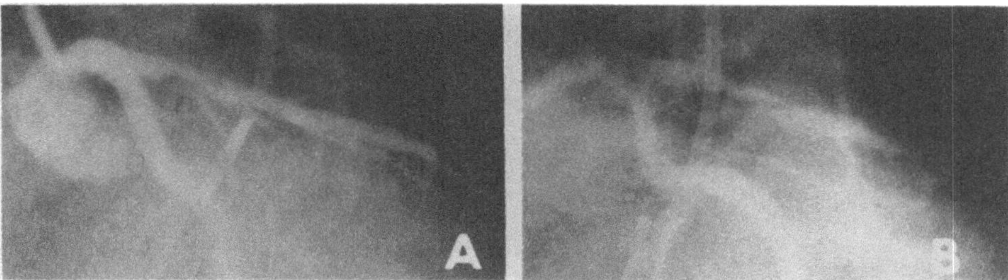

Fig. 2. A, B. Angiogram of the LAD before (A) and after (B) balloon dilatation. The initial coronary lesions characterized by marked luminal irregularities and intraluminal lucencies. After dilatation the angiographic features of dissection are visible.

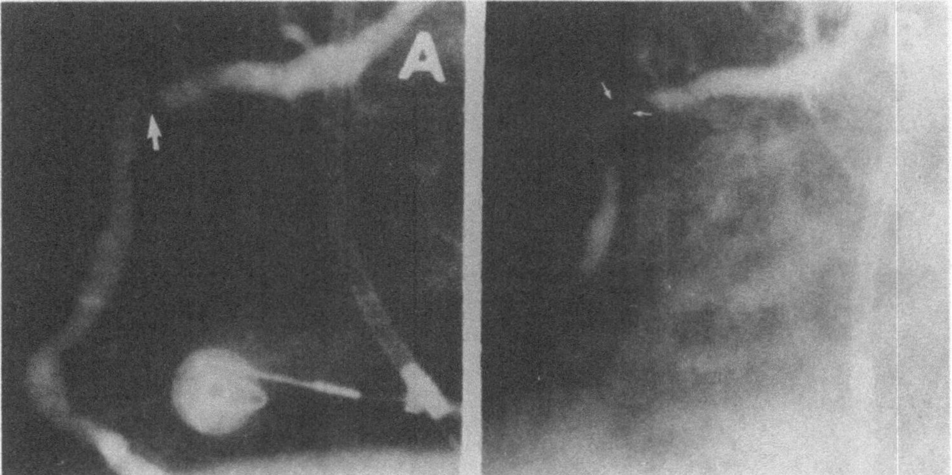

Fig. 3A, B. Angiogram of the RCA before (A) and after (B) balloon dilatation. The lesion is located at the bend of the artery (arrow, A). The column of contrast material is totally disrupted at the level of the stenosis. Dilatation resulted in occlusive coronary dissection (arrows, B). (From reference 5 with permission from Circulation)

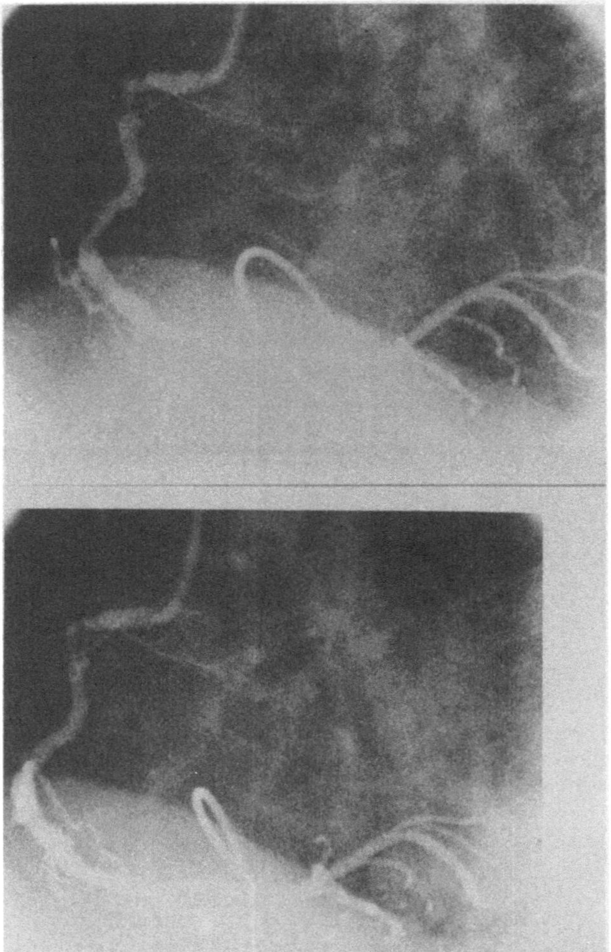

In a recent study [5] we addressed the significance of the various angiographic characteristics of coronary stenosis for the occurrence of complications due to PTCA. The angiographic criteria examined were: degree of stenosis (% diameter), length of stenosis, calcification, localization of stenosis at a vessel bifurcation, eccentricity of stenosis, localization of the stenosis in a vessel curve, irregularity of the stenosis border (Fig. 2), and intraluminal lucency (filling defect) or total disruption of flow at the level of stenosis (disruption of the column of contrast material) (Figs. 2, 3). The results of this study indicate that "complicated" lesions, in particular stenoses with border irregularity and intraluminal lucencies, as well as stenoses located in a bend of the artery (Fig. 4), may carry a significantly higher risk of occlusive coronary dissection, necessitating urgent coronary bypass surgery [5].

There are various mechanisms by which dissection and total vessel occlusion may become more likely in these situations: Atherosclerotic or thrombotic material may become more easily dislodged during crossing of a complicated plaque with the dilatation system. Plaque ulceration often involves the vessel intima and media and may result in localized weakness and decreased elasticity of the vessel wall. Creation of a false channel with the guide wire or the balloon catheter, as well as further dissection of the plaque by mechanical dilatation, appears more likely in an ulcerated lesion than in an hourglass-shaped smooth narrowing. Membrane-like transverse lesions may also carry a higher risk of iatrogenic total obstruction by mechanical irritation during the attempt to pass the lesion with the steerable guide wire. Balloon inflation within a pronounced bend of the coronary artery may enhance the "controlled" trauma to the vessel wall by generation of additional shearing forces, and does potentially increase the risk of dissection.

Earlier studies have shown that long, eccentric coronary lesions are also associated with a higher risk of coronary vascular complications and subsequent emergent surgical revascularization [2].

Eccentric coronary stenosis can often successfully be dilated; however, partial relapse of these stenoses seems to occur more often than with dilatation of concentric stenoses. This is probably due to the greater elasticity of the nondiseased segments of the dilated area, which may prevent the eccentric plaque from being effectively stretched or split. Side-branch occlusion may be another risk of PTCA if the side branch originates from the stenotic segment [6]. However, if significant side branches are at risk, double-balloon or wire + techniques may allow safe treatment of these patients [7].

The degree of stenosis is not directly related to an increase in complication rate. Mild coronary stenoses (< 60% diameter narrowing) may also carry a risk of coronary vascular complication and myocardial infarction [8]. However, the overall experience with PTCA shows that primary success seems to be lower and the complication rate somewhat higher with dilatation in tight (> 90%) stenoses. With use of the modern, low-profile balloon catheters passage of extremely tight stenoses is usually possible, and a high-grade stenotic segment [6]. However, if significant side branches are at risk, double-balloon or wire + techniques may allow safe treatment of these patients [7].

In summary, complicated angiographic morphology of coronary stenoses and localization of the stenosis in a significant bend of the artery are not contraindications of PTCA but should be taken into account when patients are selected for coronary angioplasty and informed about the chances of success and the risks of the procedure. Patients with a high clinical risk of coronary angioplasty, as described above, plus angiographic evidence of increased risk of coronary vascular complications should sometimes be denied treatment with PTCA.

The policies of patient selection for PTCA should be influenced by the experience of the angioplasty team and the conditions of the surgical stand-by. Individual and restrictive patient selection may decrease the potential pool of patients considered suitable for PTCA, but this may be acceptable in view of optimization of primary PTCA results and reduced rates of complications.

References

1. Dorros G, Cowley MJ (1985) Complications associated with PTCA. In: Ischinger T (ed) Practice of coronary angioplasty. Springer-Verlag, Berlin Heidelberg New York, pp 223–240
2. Meier B, Grüntzig AR, Hollman J, Ischinger T, Bradford JM (1983) Does length and eccentricity of coronary stenoses influence the outcome of transluminal dilatation? Circulation 67: 497–499

3. Ischinger T, Grüntzig AR (1984) Perkutane transluminale Koronarangioplastie. In Roskamm H (ed) Handbuch der inneren Medizin, Bd IX/3: Koronarerkrankungen. Springer-Verlag, Berlin Heidelberg New York, pp 1301–07

4. Levin DC, Fallon JT (1982) Significance of the angiographic morphology of localized coronary stenoses: histopathologic correlation. Circulation 66: 316–320

5. Ischinger T, Grüntzig AR, Meier B, Galan K (1986) Coronary dissection and total coronary occlusion with PTCA: significance of the initial angiographic morphology of coronary stenosis. Circulation 71

6. Meier B, Grüntzig AR, King SB, Douglas JS, Hollman J, Ischinger T, Averon F, Galan K (1984) Risk of side-branch occlusion during coronary angioplasty. Am J Cardiol 53: 10–14

7. Zack PM, Ischinger T (1984) Experience with a technique for coronary angioplasty of bifurcational lesions. Cathet Cardiovasc Diagn 10: 433–443

8. Ischinger T, Grüntzig AR, Hollman J, King SB, Douglas J, Meier B, Bradford J (1983) Should coronary arteries with less than 60% diameter stenoses be treated by angioplasty? Circulation 68: 148

9. Mabin TA, Holmes DR, Smith HC, Vlietstra RE, Bove AA, Reeder GS, Chesebro JH et al. (1985) Intracoronary thrombus: Role in coronary occlusion complicating PTCA. J Am Coll Cardiol 5: 198–202

Author's address:
Dr. T. Ischinger
Klinikum Bogenhausen
Division of Cardiology
Englschalkinger-Str. 77
8000 München 81

Obstructions Within or Immediately Adjacent to the Left Main Coronary Artery: an Indication for PTCA?

R. Simon, I. Amende, G. Herrmann, and P. R. Lichtlen

Medizinische Hochschule Hannover, Federal Republic of Germany

Introduction

Since the introduction of balloon angioplasty for coronary obstructions by Dr. Andreas Grüntzig in 1977, the indications for this procedure have progressively enlarged. Today it is well accepted that single coronary lesions as well as complex situations with multiple obstructions can be treated successfully with this innovative method. However, it is still a matter of controversy, whether or not left main coronary artery lesions should be attempted by PTCA. The data of the NHLBI registry suggest that the presence of left main coronary disease bears an increased risk for PTCA [1]. On the other hand, it has been reported that left main stem lesions can be dilated without an increase in mortality or infarction rate in selected patients [2]. Similar controversial considerations apply to balloon dilatation of very proximal stenoses of the left anterior descending artery or the left circumflex artery when the lesion is located immediately distal to the branching of the left main coronary artery, since procedure-inherent complications such as local dissection and closure may involve the main stem and thus expose the patient to a considerably increased risk. We report in this context on our experience concerning PTCA procedures in patients with left main disease or obstructions at the origin of the LAD or left circumflex artery who underwent coronary angioplasty in our institution.

Patients and methods

At the time of the collection of these data, nine patients had undergone ten PTCA procedures for left main coronary obstructions (group I) and 33 patients (group II) had had balloon angioplasty of stenoses of the LAD or the left circumflex artery located at the very origin of these vessels from the left main stem; at the same time, a total of 650 angioplasty procedures had been performed in our institution. In group I, single proximal stenoses of the MLCA were attempted in seven patients. Another patient had PTCA of a proximal left main and a sequential LAD stenosis. The remaining patient had had previous bypass surgery and patent bypass grafts to the distal LAD and a posterolateral branch of the left circumflex artery, but had an occlusion of the LAD proximal to the bypass anastomosis. This patient underwent PTCA of a severe left main stem stenosis for revascularization of the proximal LAD, which supplied a large diagonal branch and two large septal branches. In addition, an obstructed bypass graft to the right coronary artery was dilated during the same procedure. PTCA of the left main coronary artery was repeated in this patient because of recurrence of the stenosis after the first procedure.

In group II, 24 of the 33 patients had PTCA of proximal LAD lesions that were located adjacent to the MLCA branching (an example is given in Fig. 1). In seven patients obstructions of the LAD origin and, in addition, of the mid LAD and/or diagonal branches or septal branches were attempted. The remaining two patients underwent PTCA for stenoses at the LAD origin and in the mid circumflex artery, or at the circumflex origin and in the mid LAD, respectively.

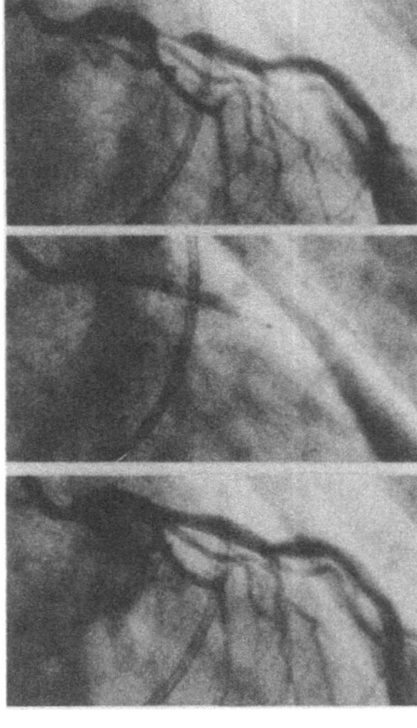

Fig. 1. Angioplasty of a stenosis at the LAD origin.

Balloon catheter systems with steerable guide wires were used in the majority of cases. Since the balloon had to be inflated in the left main coronary artery in all patients, an increased extent of ischemia was anticipated; therefore, pulmonary wedge pressure as an estimate of left ventricular filling pressure was continuously monitored in conjunction with aortic pressure, distal coronary pressure, and the electrocardiogram in all patients throughout the procedure. In group I, coronary sinus blood flow was continuously recorded during balloon inflation in an attempt to monitor more closely changes in left ventricular perfusion during the ischemic phase.

Results

MLCA Obstructions

Primary success (defined in our institution as a > 30% increase in vessel luminal diameter and resulting in a residual stenosis of < 50%) was achieved in six of the nine patients in group I. It is of interest that balloon inflation time could be prolonged to 1 min and more in most cases, although the balloon blocked the entire inflow to the left coronary system (Fig. 2). All six patients underwent control angiography 3–6 months after the procedure. Four had a persistent good result (example in Fig. 3), whereas two patients had recurrence of the stenosis; this was severe in one patient, who underwent successful redilatation. The other patient had moderate recurrence 3 months later (about 50% luminal obstruction) and was treated medically, but 1 year later the stenosis had progressed to more than 70% in diameter obstruction and he underwent elective bypass surgery.
In two patients the MLCA stenosis could not be dilated. In both, an eccentric obstruction of the vessel was present. A 3.7-mm balloon could be fully inflated at rather low pressures (2–3 bar) but left the stenosis completely unaltered (Fig. 4).
In the remaining patient, a tight proximal stenosis of the left main coronary artery was dilated successfully. Ten minutes after the completely uneventful procedure, the final coronary angiogram demonstrated a proximal occlusion of the LAD that had developed

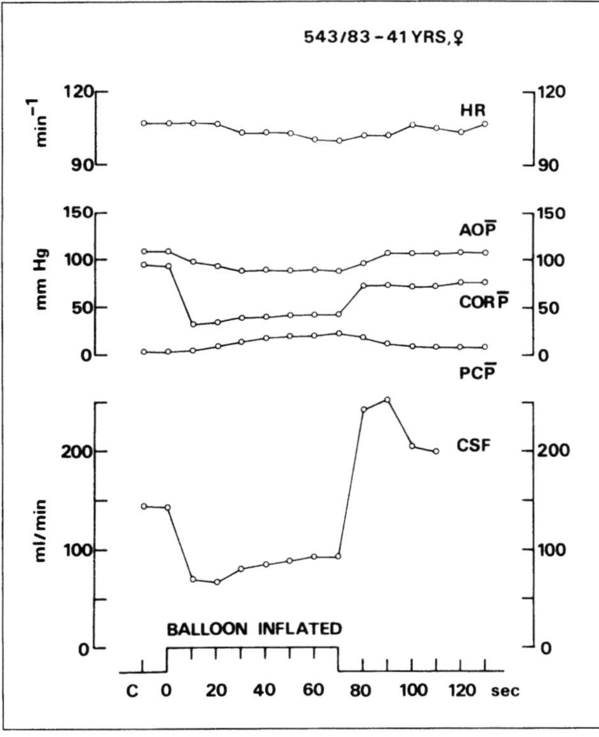

Fig. 2. Hemodynamic events during balloon inflation in a 41-year-old female patient undergoing PTCA of a proximal stenosis in the left main coronary artery. HR, heart rate; AOP̄, mean aortic pressure; CORP̄, distal coronary pressure; PCP̄, mean pulmonary capillary wedge pressure; CSF, coronary sinus blood flow (thermodilution technique).

PTCA OF THE LEFT MAIN CORONARY ARTERY
♂, 53 YRS (263/82)

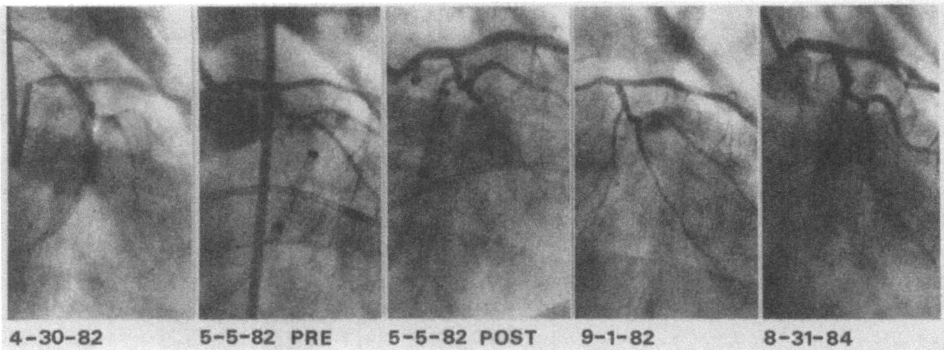

Fig. 3. Early and late results after PTCA of a left main coronary artery lesion in a 53-year-old male patient with unstable angina pectoris. Coronary angiograms are shown 5 days before (4/30/82), immediately before (5/5/82 PRE), and after successful angioplasty (5/5/82 POST), at early follow-up (9/1/82), and at late follow-up (8/31/84) 27 months later.

UNSUCCESSFUL PTCA OF A MLCA OBSTRUCTION
♂, 52 YRS, UNSTABLE ANGINA (42/85)

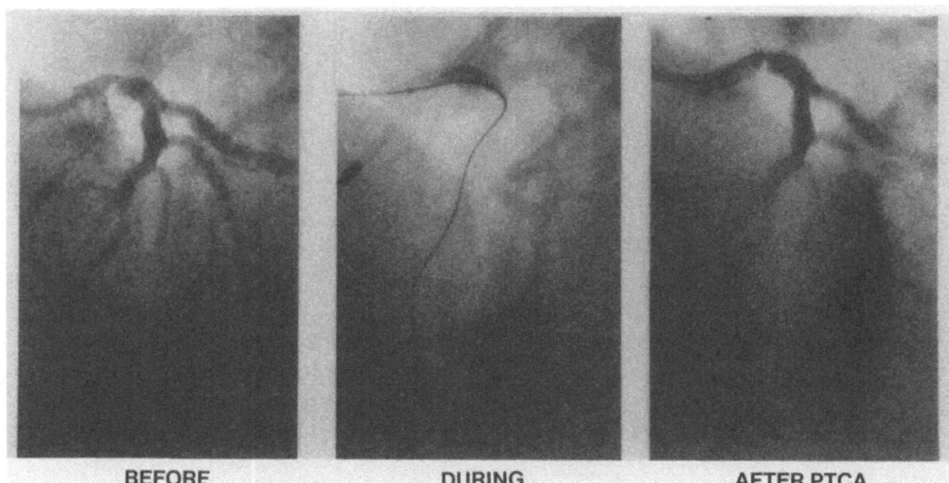

Fig. 4. Unsuccessful attempt of a left main coronary obstruction in a 52-year-old male patient with unstable angina pectoris.

104

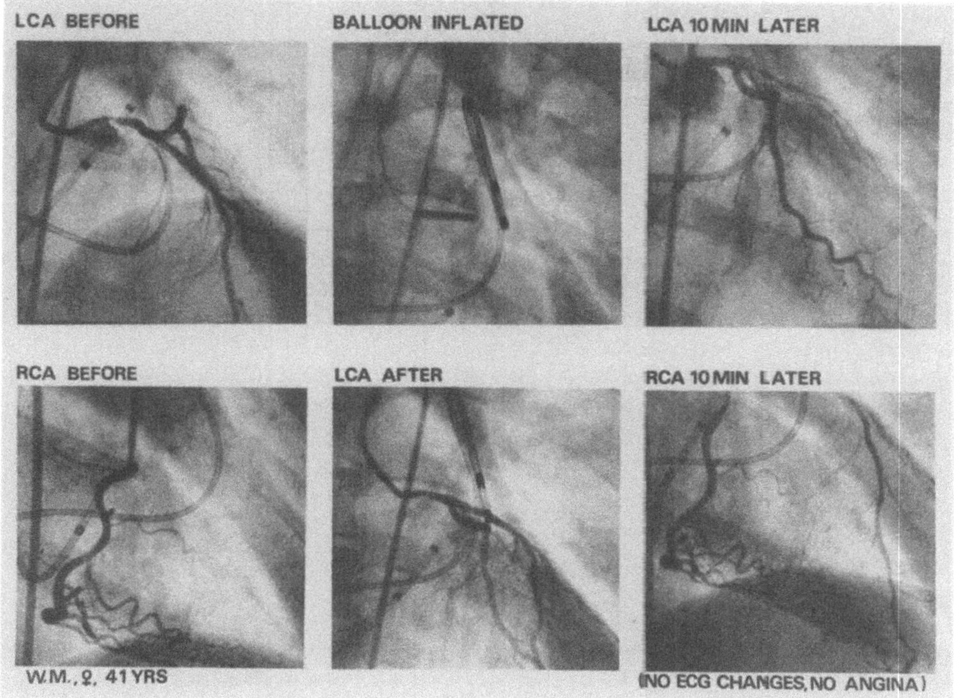

Fig. 5. Development of a proximal LAD occlusion after a primarily successful dilatation of an MLCA obstruction, associated with rapid development of collateral filling in a 41-year-old female patient. Left: angiogram of the left and right coronary artery before dilation. Note the absence of collaterals to the left coronary system. Middle: balloon inflated in the left main obstruction and result after dilatation. Right: asymptomatic proximal occlusion of the LAD 10 min later (above), associated with a rapid collateral perfusion from the right coronary artery (below) that had not been present before the procedure.

without any chest pain and in the presence of a completely normal electrocardiogram and pulmonary wedge pressure. Contrast injection into the right coronary artery revealed a rapid collateral filling of the entire LAD, that had not been present before the dilatation (see Fig. 5). This patient underwent immediate bypass surgery. There were no other operations, no myocardial infarctions, no deaths, and no further complications in group-I patients.

Obstructions of the LAD or Circumflex Origin

Among the 33 patients with very proximal LAD or circumflex obstructions in group II, primary success was achieved in 30 (90%) and partial success (reduction of the diameter obstruction from 90% to 60%) was seen in another patient. Twenty-seven of these 31 patients underwent angiographic restudy. Twenty (74%) showed a persistent good result 3–6 months after the procedure, whereas seven (26%) had recurrence of the stenosis.

The extension of an intimal tear originating from the site of the dilated stenosis into the left main coronary artery was observed in four cases of group II. This did not cause any problem in three patients, but it led to a dissection of the MLCA in the fourth patient; this was followed by thrombus formation and subsequent total occlusion of the left main coronary artery, associated with cardiogenic shock. The immediate recrossing and dilatation of the MLCA opened the vessel and allowed the percutaneous insertion of an aortic counterpulsation balloon under stable circulatory conditions. The patient underwent immediate bypass surgery and had an uneventful postoperative course, but the electrocardiogram showed an anterior myocardial infarction after operation. Another patient underwent emergency surgery because of a proximal occlusion of the LAD at the site of the dilatation, which could be recrossed repeatedly but continued to close despite multiple attempts. There were no further complications and no deaths in group II; the rate of emergency bypass surgery was 2/33 patients (6%), the infarction rate 1/33 patients (3%).

Comment

There are few reports in the literature concerning balloon angioplasty for left main coronary obstructions. Grüntzig [3] mentioned two cases in his initial report on PTCA in 1978, one of them successful. In another early report, Kaltenbach et al. [4] desribed angioplasty for MLCA disease in three patients; it was successful in two, but failed in the third. Stertzer et al. [2] reported PTCA for left main obstructions in eight patients with multivessel disease, with primary success in all patients and a recurrence rate of 25%. They concluded that "despite concern, PTCA of the MLCA is feasible without increased risk in selected cases." Dorros et al. [5] have reported similarly favorable results in five patients with multivessel disease.

In the largest series so far on PTCA for MLCA disease, Biamino et al. [6] reported a primary success rate of 78% in 32 patients, most of them with multivessel disease and having had previous bypass surgery. The in-hospital mortality in their series, however, amounted to 6%. To our knowledge, experiences with angioplasty for severe obstructions of the LAD or circumflex origin have not been reported in a collected series. Our current experience seems to support the view that lesions in the proximal left main coronary artery itself and in the immediate vicinity of the left main branching can be attempted by PTCA in selected cases, with an acceptable risk and a rate of success that is comparable to the well-known results for more distal sites. In case of vascular complications, however, the operator has to be prepared for more serious and dramatic events than with more distal dilatations. We have therefore restricted angioplasty for left main lesions to selected patients with small circumflex arteries and dominant and unconspicuous right coronary arteries, in order to reduce the potential risk of complications. Furthermore, special precautions are taken during PTCA of MLCA stenoses as well as of lesions of the origin of the LAD or left circumflex artery. These precautions include extended hemodynamic monitoring during the procedure, the preparation of both groins to allow rapid installation of aortic counterpulsation in case of complications, and a surgical stand-by with an operating room nearby and the immediate availability of a surgical team.

106

References

1. Dorros G, Cowley M, Janke L, Kelsey SF, Mullen SM, van Raden M (1984) In-hospital mortality rate in the National Heart, Lung and Blood Institute percutaneous transluminal coronary angioplasty registry. Am J Cardiol 53: 17C
2. Stertzer SH, Wallsh E, Bruno MS (1981) Evaluation of transluminal coronary angioplasty in left main coronary artery stenosis. Am J Cardiol 47: 396
3. Grüntzig A (1978) Transluminal dilatation of coronary artery stenosis. Lancet I: 263
4. Kaltenbach M, Kober G, Scherer D (1980) Mechanische Dilatation von Koronarstenosen (transluminale Angioplastie). Z Kardiol 69: 1
5. Dorros G, Stertzer SH, Cowley J, Myler RK (1984) Complex coronary angioplasty: multiple coronary dilatations. Am J Cardiol 53: 126C
6. Biamino G, Hartzler GO, Rutherfold BD, McConhahay DR, Johnson WL (1985) Left main coronary PTCA is a reasonable palliative procedure. J Am Coll Cardiol 5: 520

Authors' address:
Dr. R. Simon
Medizinische Hochschule Hannover
Zentrum Innere Medizin
Karl-Wiechert-Allee
3000 Hannover

Recanalization of Totally Occluded Coronary Vessels by Percutaneous Transluminal Coronary Angioplasty

R. Erbel, C. Diefenbach, G. Schreiner, T. Pop, C. von Olshausen,
H. J. Rupprecht, A. Aydin, and J. Meyer

II. Medical Clinic, Johannes Gutenberg-University, Mainz,
Federal Republic of Germany

Introduction

Since its introduction in 1977, percutaneous transluminal coronary angioplasty (PTCA)
has become an effective approach for treatment of patients with single-vessel disease
[1–3, 5]. Treatment of double- and multiple-vessel disease has also been attempted [5, 6].
In patients with angina pectoris total occlusion of coronary vessels is found, and PTCA
has also been used in an attempt to restore coronary blood flow in such patients [8, 10].
Even main stem occlusions have been recanalized [11]. In patients with total occlusion of
coronary vessels, collateral flow is sufficient to maintain cardiac function at rest but not
during exercise [12–14]. Therefore, PTCA seems to be an ideal method for restoring antegrade coronary blood flow.
This report presents the results of recanalization performed in our catheterization laboratory between January 1983 and August 1985. Technical aspects, success rate, and follow-
up data are given.

Methods

Patient Selection

From January 1983 to August 1985 PTCA was attempted, with written informed consent, in 38 patients with total coronary artery occlusion. These 38 patients represent 8%
of all patients who underwent PTCA during this period in the catheterization laboratory
of the II Medical Clinic in Mainz.
Diagnostic coronary angiography showed a relevant significant stenosis in 22 of the 225
patients (10%, Fig. 1). At the time of PTCA the coronary artery was occluded without development of acute myocardial infarction because of recruitable collateral vessels. The
time interval between the diagnostic procedure and PTCA ranged from 13 days to 6
months; the mean was 77 days. Total coronary occlusion of one vessel, found in 16 patients at the time of the diagnostic coronary angiography, was thought to be suitable for
PTCA. Nineteen patients were in stable angina and 19 in unstable angina. Main stem
coronary artery occlusion was found in one patient suffering from evolving myocardial
infarction. Eighteen patients had single-vessel disease, ten patients had double- and nine
patients three-vessel disease, but the second luminal narrowing was not more than 70%.

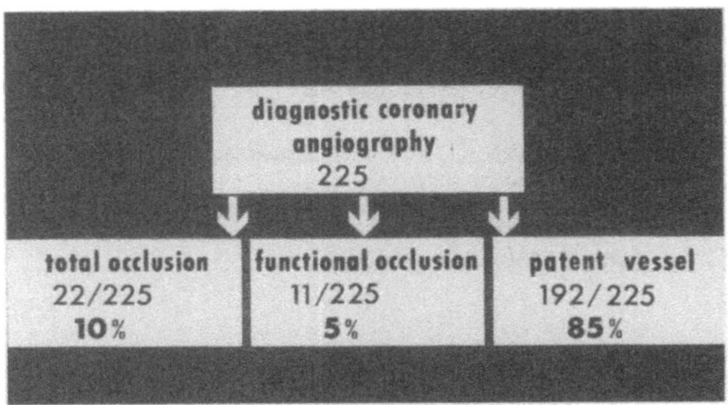

Fig. 1. Results of diagnostic outside coronary angiography in 225 patients and the control coronary angiography before PTCA in our institution.

The occluded vessel was the left anterior descending coronary artery in 21 patients, the right coronary artery in 11 patients, and the left circumflex coronary artery in four patients. One main stem occlusion and one coronary bypass occlusion were treated.

Recanalization was performed only in patients with good collateral flow (score II-III), when the distal part of the occluded coronary vessel had been filled by the collaterals; i.e. recanalization was not attempted in the case of an occlusion directly at the origin of a vessel if the first part of the vessel was not visualized.

The time of occlusion could be estimated in only 20 patients for whom previous coronary angiograms were available and in whom new symptoms had occurred. In the other patients, the time from the first to the second coronary angiography was known.

Treatment

PTCA was performed as previously described [4]. The catheters used are listed in Table 1. In two patients, a 3-F recanalization catheter (Schneider Medintag) was used first for

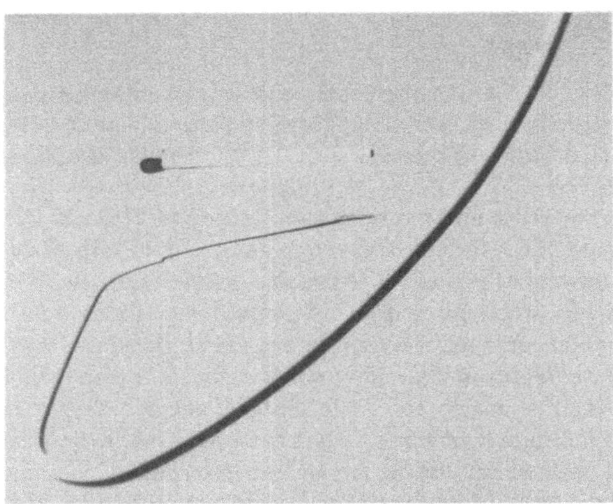

Fig. 2. A 3-F recanalization catheter imaged after introduction through a 7-F Judkins catheter

Table 1. Catheters used for successful recanalization in 19 patients with total coronary occlusion

No. of patients	Catheter type
2	3-F recanalization
3	G 20-20 Grüntzig
5	G 20-20 Grüntzig
3	Double balloon
2	DG 20-30
3	3.0 steerable
3	Hartzler 2.0, 2.5

restoring coronary blood flow (Fig. 2). After recanalization, balloon catheters could be introduced.

Nitrates and calcium antagonists were administered during each procedure to prevent coronary spasm. Success was defined as an improvement in the stenosis by 20% or more of luminal diameter.

Results

A typical example of recanalization of an occluded coronary artery is shown in Fig. 3. When the left coronary angiogram was performed, collaterals to the right coronary artery could be seen. The right coronary artery was occluded, but after recanalization it was patent and without residual lesions, and the collaterals had disappeared. The stress test and thallium scintigrams had been positive before PTCA but were negative after the procedure.

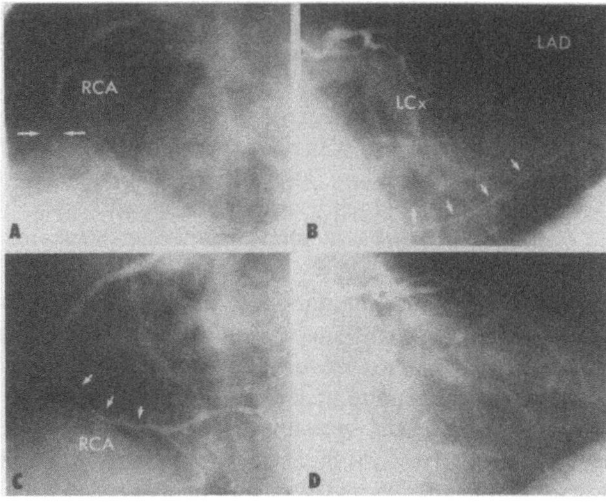

Fig. 3. a) Occluded right coronary artery (RCA) b) Collateral flow (arrows) to the right coronary artery c) After recanalization antegrade flow in the right coronary artery without residual lesions d) Left coronary artery, collaterals disappeared.

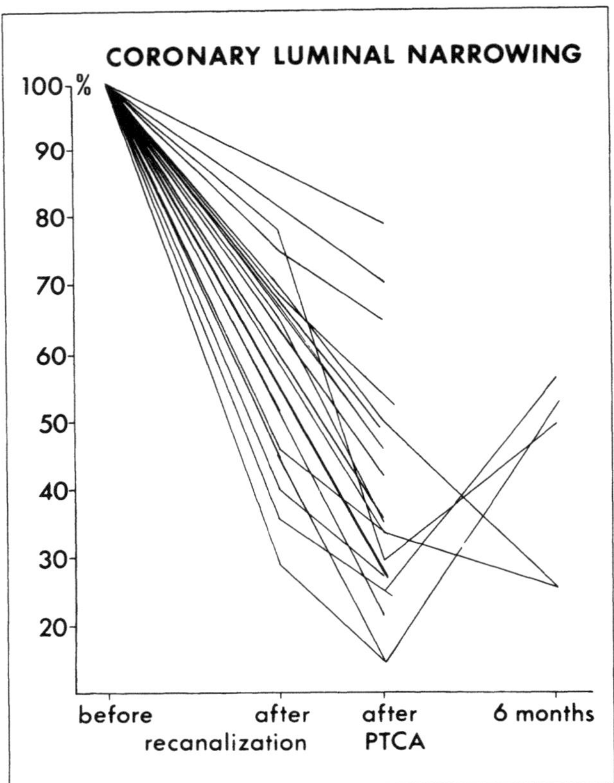

Fig. 4. Area stenosis of patients with successful recanalization of coronary arteries (n = 19).

The results of the recanalization of occluded coronary vessels are illustrated in Fig. 4. Recanalization was successful in 19/38 patients (50%). Various types of catheters were used for recanalization (Table 1), and there was no clear advantage with any one type. The recanalization catheters had the advantage of allowing the use of steel guide wires by which the catheters could be advanced more easily. After recanalization balloon catheters were used.

Recanalization was successful in 21 patients (43%) with occlusion of the left anterior descending coronary artery, in eight of 11 patients (73%) with right coronary artery occlusion, in one patient with left main stem occlusion, and in one patient with a bypass occlusion. The luminal narrowing of the coronary arteries before and after the procedure is illustrated in Fig. 4. Collaterals disappeared immediately after recanalization in all patients.

Signs of chest discomfort appeared with ECG changes in nine successfully recanalized patients and CPK changes in five. Of the 19 patients with unsuccessful recanalization (Fig. 5) 10 underwent coronary bypass surgery and nine were treated medically within six months. Another one from the medically treated group underwent coronary bypass surgery within a year. Of the 19 patients with successful recanalization, 17 were medically treated and two underwent coronary bypass surgery within 6 months. Another two from the medically treated group underwent coronary bypass surgery within 12 months.

112

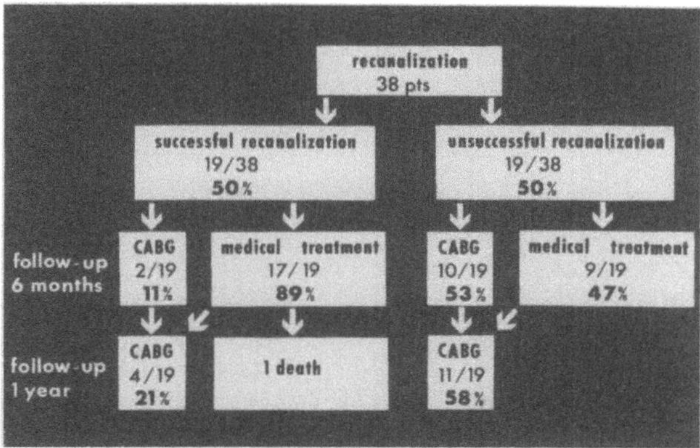

Fig. 5. Results and follow-up in 38 patients with recanalization of coronary arteries.

Discussion

Percutaneous transluminal coronary angioplasty (PTCA) has become a safe procedure in patients with single-vessel disease [1–7]. The success rate has increased from 70% to nearly 90% in highly selected groups. Treatment of multiple-vessel disease has also been attempted successfully [6, 7].

In about 10% of patients selected for PTCA complete occlusion of the coronary artery is found between the diagnostic procedure and the PTCA [10]. Our results are in accordance with these findings. Progression of coronary artery stenosis is slow and unpredictable, but the most severe stenosis has the greatest tendency to progress, often to complete occlusion [9]. Even occlusion of the left main stem has been observed [11].

Occlusion of the coronary artery seems to be silent in patients with development of collateral flow, maintaining regional myocardial function during rest. During exercise collateral flow usually is not sufficient to prevent coronary insufficiency [12–14]. Therefore, restoration of antegrade blood flow seems to be a logical step to relieve angina in these patients. Success rates for recanalization of occluded coronary arteries range from 45% [9] to 71% [15]. Table 2 lists the results reported by several authors. Success seems to be dependent on the site of the lesion, as our results demonstrate, but occlusion time is a major factor [8]. In patients with occlusion times longer than 12 weeks no vessel could be recanalized [8].

Table 2. Success rates and restenosis rates found in the literature

Reference	n	Success rate (%)	Restenosis rate (%)	
Dervan et al. 1983	13	54	43	(24)
Stürzenhofecker 1983	14	71	–	–
Schreiner 1984	14	65	–	–
Serruys et al. 1985	49	57	40	
		–45 totally occluded		
		–81 functionally occluded		
Holmes et al. 1984	24	54	20	–
Erbel 1986	38	50		

In patients in whom balloon catheters fail, smaller recanalization catheters can be used, followed after restoration of coronary blood flow by PTCA.

In 25% of our patients chest discomfort was observed, as previously reported [8, 9], possibly related to peripheral embolization. However, coronary angiography provided no evidence for this event.

After restoration of antegrade coronary flow, collaterals disappeared immediately, as previously described for a patient with main stem occlusion [11].

Holmes et al. [8] reported a recurrence rate of 20% and Dervan et al. [16] of 41%. The restenosis rate seems to be somewhat higher than in usual PTCA candidates, possibly related to different intrinsic vascular and hematologic propensities for acute occlusion of existing arteriosclerotic lesions, or to the more pronounced pathological rupture of the vessel wall through the longitudinal shearing of the arteriosclerotic and fibrocellular material [9].

In conclusion, PTCA is a safe technique for restoring antegrade blood flow in occluded coronary arteries. The success rate is dependent on occlusion time. Relief of symptoms can be found, but there is a high recurrence rate. A routine check after 6 months is necessary to monitor patients' therapy.

References

1. Grüntzig AR, Senning A, Siegenthaler WE (1979) Nonoperative dilatation of coronary artery stenosis: percutaneous transluminal coronary angioplasty. N Engl J Med 301: 61–68
2. Grüntzig AR (1984) Percutaneous transluminal coronary angioplasty: 6 years' experience. Am Heart J 107: 818–823
3. Meyer J, Böcker B, Erbel R, Bardos P, Messmer BJ, Effert S (1980) Treatment of unstable angina with transluminal coronary angioplasty (PTCA). Circulation 62/III: 160 (abstr)
4. Meyer J, Schmitz H, Erbel R, Kiesslich T, Böcker-Josephs B, Krebs W, Braun PC, Bardos P, Minale C, Messmer BJ, Effert S (1981) Treatment of unstable angina pectoris with percutaneous transluminal coronary angioplasty. Cathet Cardiovasc Diagn 7: 361–371
5. Williams DO, Riley RS, Singh AK, Gewirtz H, Most RS (1981) Evaluation of the role of coronary angioplasty in patients with unstable angina pectoris. Am Heart J 102: 1–9
6. Hartzler GO (1983) Percutaneous transluminal coronary angioplasty in multivessel disease. Cathet Cardiovasc Diagn 9: 537–542
7. Dorros G, Stertzer SH, Cowley MJ, Myler RK (1984) Complex Coronary angioplasty: multiple coronary dilatations. AM J Cardiol 53: 126–130
8. Holmes DR jr, Vlietstra RE, Reeder GS, Bresnahan JF, Smith HC, Bove AA, Schaff HV (1984) Angioplasty in total coronary artery occlusion T Am Coll Cardiol 3: 845–849
9. Serruys PW, Umans V, Heyndrickx GR, v. d. Brand M, De Feyter PJ, Wijns W, Jaski B, Hugenholtz PG (1985) Elective PTCA of totally occluded coronary arteries not associated with acute myocardial infarction; short-term and long-term results. Eur Heart Journal 6: 2–12
10. Kober G, Hopf R, Reinemer H, Kaltenbach M (1985) Langzeitergebnisse der transluminalen koronaren Angioplastie von chronischen Herzkranzgefäßverschlüssen. Z Kardiol 74: 309–316
11. Erbel R, Meinertz T, Wessler I, Meyer J, Seybold-Epting (1984) Recanalization of occluded left main coronary artery in unstable angina pectoris. Am J Cardiol 53: 1725–1727
12. Kolibash AJ, Bush CA, Wepsic RA, Schroeder DP, Tetalman MR, Lewis RP (1982) Coronary collateral vessels: spectrum of physiologic capabilities with respect to providing rest and stress myocardial perfusion, maintenance or left ventricular function and protection against infarction. Am J Cardiol 50: 230–238
13. Giorgi LV, Hartzler GO, Rutherford BD, McConahay DR (1983) Angina following total coronary occlusion: definitive treatment with percutaneous coronary angioplasty. J Am Coll Cardiol 1: 656

14. Eng C, Paterson RE, Horowitz SF, et al (1982) Coronary collateral function during exercise. Circulation 66: 309–316
15. Stürzenhofecker P (1983) Transluminale mechanische Rekanalisierung mit Angioplastie total verschlossener Coronararterien. Morphologische und funktionelle Ergebnisse. Z Kardiol 72: 65
16. Dervan JP, Baim DS, Cherniles J, Grossman (1983) Transluminal angioplasty of occluded coronary arteries: use of a movable guide wire system. Circulation 68: 776–784
17. Schreiner G, Erbel R, Pop T, Meyer J (1984) Mechanische Rekanalisation von totalen Koronarverschlüssen. Z f Kardiol 73, Suppl. 1 : 34

Authors' address:
Prof. Dr. med. Raimund Erbel
II. Medical Clinic
Johannes Gutenberg University
Langenbeckstr. 1
D-6500 Mainz
Federal Republic of Germany

Percutaneous Transluminal Coronary Angioplasty in Acute Myocardial Infarction With and Without Prior Systemic Fibrinolytic Therapy

W. Rutsch M. Schartl, and H. Schmutzler

Klinikum Charlottenburg of the Free University of Berlin, Federal Republic of Germany, Department of Cardiology

Since its introduction by Grüntzig in 1977, percutaneous transluminal coronary angioplasty (PTCA) has been applied to patients with symptomatic coronary artery disease. Although the technique was initially practiced in patients with stable angina, experience has shown that it may be applied in patients with unstable angina and acute myocardial infarction, with and without prior fibrinolytic therapy, as well. During acute myocardial infarction, intracoronary infusion of streptokinase can open 70%–90% of acutely obstructed coronary arteries. However, in most patients, residual high-grade atheromatous lesions remain at the site of occlusion, with a potential for continued myocardial ischemia, unstable angina, coronary reocclusion, and reinfarction. Consequently, mechanical interventions such as CABG or PTCA may be required after thrombolytic therapy. On the other hand, PTCA can be used as definitive therapy for coronary artery recanalization in acute evolving myocardial infarction, if complications arising from thrombolytic therapy would exclude the patient from an acute recanalization procedure. We describe our clinical experience with PTCA after intravenous streptokinase (SK) and as primary therapy in the management of patients with acute myocardial infarction.

Sixty men and ten women underwent emergency cardiac catheterization during the first 3 h after the onset of chest pain and ST elevation consistent with acute myocardial infarction. Their ages ranged from 23 to 77 years, with a mean age of 52 ± 10 years.

The infarct-related vessel was the LAD in 41% of cases, the RCA in 57%, and the circumflex artery or its branches in 2%. Eighty-one percent of patients had single-vessel disease, 13% two-vessel disease, and 6% three-vessel disease. Collaterals to the infarct-related vessel were demonstrated in 19% of cases. Six patients were in cardiogenic shock and seven had third-degree AV block. Patients referred from other hospitals were given 1 million IU of SK intravenously over 30 min as soon as the diagnosis of infarction was made, while patients from our hospital were transported immediately to the catheterization laboratory. Group I comprised 43 patients who had received SK, and group II was made up of 27 patients who underwent PTCA without prior SK infusion.

After patients' arrival in the catheterization laboratory, a single-plane ventriculogram and coronary angiograms of both vessels were made using the Judkins technique. The occluded vessel was identified and PTCA was performed with a steerable guide-wire system.

Patients in group II without systemic SK therapy received 10000 IU of heparin by bolus injection. Following PTCA, patients received a continuous infusion of nifedipine or nitroglycerine, and oral anticoagulation with dicoumarol was administered during the hospital phase. After discharge, the drug regimen included 250 mg acetylicsalicylic acid and 10 mg nifedipine three times daily. Bicycle ergometry, thallium scintigraphy, and follow-up angiographic studies were made before discharge. Depending on these results, medical therapy was continued or a second PTCA or bypass surgery was performed (see Table 1).

Unfavourable vascular relations such as tortuosity (Fig. 1), severe diffuse coronary artery disease, or an extremely peripheral site of occlusion prevented mechanical dilatation in 6% (n = 4). In 9% of patients we had different technical problems: It was impossible to place the guide wire in a correct position distal to the occlusion, or permanent recanalization could not be maintained, even though the position of the balloon catheter was correct. Where unfavorable vascular relations made PTCA impracticable, intracoronary administration of SK was employed. No complications were observed in 81% of patients undergoing PTCA. Local dissection occurred without sequelae in 6% of patients, and dissection with subsequent occlusion was observed in 6% of cases. Emergency CABG was performed in two patients (3%); PTCA resulted in temporary reperfusion followed by reocclusion in one patient, while occlusion of the circumflex artery supervened in one pa-

Table 1. Sequence of treatment for patients in groups I and II

1. Group I – streptokinase intravenous, 1 million U/30 min
2. Group II – no streptokinase, heparin 10 000 U
3. Ventriculogram
4. Coronary angiogram
5. Percutaneous transluminal coronary angioplasty
6. Unsuccessful PTCA: intracoronary streptokinase
7. Anticoagulation (heparin, dicoumarol), infusion of nifedipine oder nitroglycerine
8. Third week: bicycle ergometry, thallium scan, coronary angiogram, ventriculogram
9. Medical therapy, second PTCA or CABG

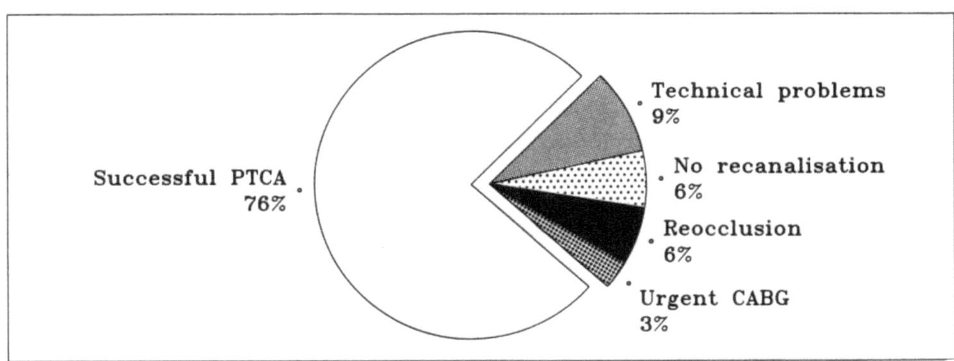

Fig. 1. Results of PTCA in 70 patients with acute myocardial infarction

118

tient with proximal occlusion of the LAD and a short left main stem; it may be that thrombotic material was dislodged from the LAD. Both patients survived coronary bypass surgery without complications and with good functional results.

Perforation of the occlusion and ballon dilatation were judged successful when residual stenosis was less than 50%. PTCA was successful in 85% (n = 60) of cases according to this criterion. Residual stenosis immediately after PTCA was 45% ± 11% in patients of group I with preliminary systemic SK infusion and 39% ± 15% at angiographic follow-up 3 weeks later (Fig. 2). This compares with residual stenosis of 41% ± 16% immediately after PTCA and 36% ± 14% 3 weeks later in patients in group II, without prior fibrinolytic therapy. Four patients in group II had contraindications to treatment with SK – recent gastric ulcer in two cases and thorax trauma secondary to cardiopulmonary resuscitation in two others. Both of the latter were in cardiogenic shock and demonstrated prompt improvement after mechanical recanalization. A mean of 12 ± 8 min elapsed between demonstration of the occluded vessel, decision to perform mechanical dilatation and successful completion of PTCA. In comparison, combined systemic and intracoronary administration of SK averaged 19 ± 11 min until reperfusion was achieved.

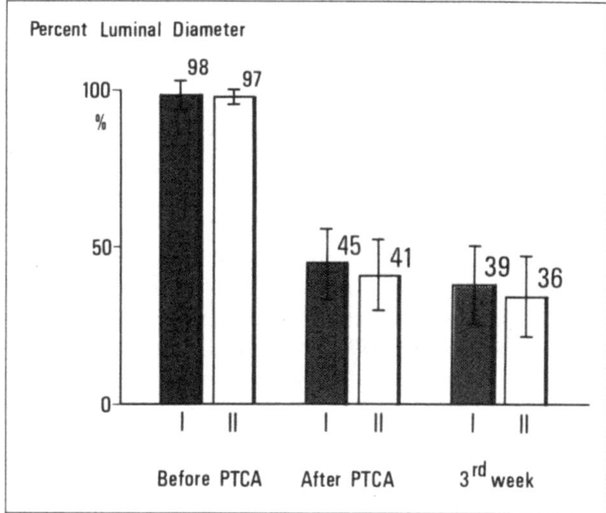

Fig. 2. Success of PTCA according to extent of residual stenosis in 70 patients

Repeat PTCA was carried out in 9% of patients who demonstrated restenosis at follow-up. Two others (4%) suffered reocclusion with chest pain and ST elevation, on the 4th and 7th day respectively; repeat PTCA was successful in both cases. One patient suffered reocclusion without reinfarction. Sudden cardiac death occurred in one patient during the 3rd week after successful PTCA. The remaining 85% of patients with initially successful PTCA were free of ischemic events during the hospital phase (Fig. 3).

Ultimate extent of infarction correlates with left ventricular function, early and late mortality, and arrhythmias. One of the most important objectives in treatment of acute evol-

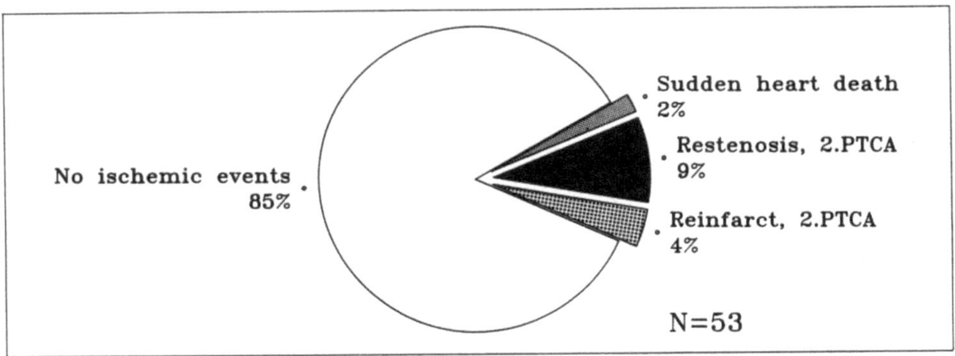

Fig. 3. Results of in-hospital follow-up after successful PTCA in 53 patients

ving myocardial infarction is limitation of infarct size. Re-establishment of myocardial perfusion by recanalization of the occluded vessel is the most important factor in this effort. Although intracoronary infusion of SK is capable of achieving recanalization in a large percentage of cases, especially when combined with preliminary intravenous SK infusion, most patients have significant residual stenosis at the end of the procedure. This limits adequate myocardial reperfusion, and the degree of stenosis correlates directly with the reocclusion rate. Since reocclusion occurs most often in the first few days after fibrinolytic recanalization, and functional improvement cannot be determined quantitatively, PTCA would appear to be superior to CABG. Optimal reperfusion is achieved early, and the reocclusion rate is low. Initial success rates are high, and there are few complications. In summary, one may conclude that PTCA, both with and without preliminary intravenous SK infusion, offers significant advantages over intracoronary administration of SK in the treatment of evolving myocardial infarction. Adequate reperfusion is achieved within a shorter period of time, the reocclusion rate is lower, and ischemic events occur less frequently in the early follow-up period. When contraindications to fibrinolytic therapy are present, PTCA and anticoagulation may be the only measures available for achieving recanalization. PTCA is an attractive alternative to fibrinolytic therapy and early or late CABG in patients with acute myocardial infarction.

References

1. Hartzler G et al. (1983) Percutaneous transluminal coronary angioplasty with and without thrombolytic therapy for treatment of acute myocardial infarction. Am Heart J 106: 965-973
2. Hartzler G, Rutherford B, McConohay (1984) Percutaneous transluminal coronary angioplasty: application for acute myocardial infarction. Am J Cardiol 53: 117C-121C
3. Papapietro S et al (1985) Percutaneous transluminal coronary angioplasty after intracoronary streptokinase in evolving acute myocardial infarction. Am J Cardiol 55: 48-53
4. Serruys P et al (1983) Is transluminal coronary angioplasty mandatory after successful thrombolysis? Quantitative coronary angiographic study. Br Heart J 50: 257-265

5. Gold H et al (1984) combined intracoronary streptokinase infusion and coronary angioplasty during acute myocardial infarction. Am J Cardiol 53: 122C-125C
6. Pepine C, et al (1984) Percutaneous transluminal coronary angioplasty immediately after intracoronary streptolysis of transmural myocardial infarction. Circulation 66 (5): 905-913
8. Meyer J et al (1984) Transluminale Angioplastie – unstabile Angina, frischer Infarkt. Z Kardiol 73 (2): 167-176
9. Meyer J, et al (1985) Sequential intervention procedures after intracoronary thrombolysis; balloon dilatation, bypass surgery, and medical treatment. Int J Cardiol 7: 281-293

Authors' address:
Dr. W. Rutsch
Klinikum Charlottenburg
der Freien Universität Berlin.
Spandauer Damm 130
1000 Berlin 19

The Follow-up of PTCA Using Thallium-201 Myocardial Scintigraphy

C.-M. Kirsch

Siemens Gammasonics Inc., Des Plaines, USA

Myocardial scintigraphy applying the potassium analog thallium (Tl) 201 has become a routine method in nuclear cardiology using planar gamma camera imaging in various projections. It is usually carried out in two imaging sessions, the first performed immediately after maximal exercise to depict stress-induced ischemia and the second after 3 or 4 h to show the Tl 201 distribution at rest. It provides a high sensitivity (83%) and specificity (90%) in the detection of patients with coronary heart disease (CHD) [1]. Therefore, it has been used to monitor patients after therapy since the late 1970s [2-4]. Planar imaging, however, is hampered by the superimposition of myocardial and surrounding structures, thus allowing accurate judgement only for structures that project unequivocally, such as the anterior wall.

The introduction of tomographic imaging techniques (single photon emission computed tomography, SPECT) provides a three-dimensional display of all myocardial areas without any superimposition, thus allowing a more precise assessment of the state of the myocardium [5]. In a recent study the usefulness and advantages of Tl 201 SPECT in the detection of patients with CHD could be demonstrated [6, 7]. As a consequence, this imaging technique was also applied in the follow-up of patients after PTCA.

Instrumentation

SPECT was performed by means of rotating gamma camera systems. The gamma camera is mounted on a gantry in a tunnel configuration, allowing rotation of the camera head around the patient, who is in a supine position on a couch. Two instruments were used for our examinations: a single-head, large-field-of-view gamma camera equipped with a high-resolution parallel-hole collimator (CGR, Gammatome 9000) and a dual-head camera system with low-energy all-purpose (LEAP) collimators (Siemens, ROTA camera), both on line to a dedicated computer system. The projection images were recorded as 64 × 64 matrices on either instrument with 64 or 60 angular projections over 360°. The single-head instrument used continuous rotation as compared with the ROTA camera in step and shoot mode. The time for data acquisition was 22 min in either case. Thereafter, the transverse slices on both machines were reconstructed by filtered back-projection without attenuation correction and a subsequent calculation of the sagittal, frontal, or oblique-frontal planes.

Patients

Our patient population comprised a total of 53 individuals with CHD, all of whom were studied before and after PTCA. Each patient exercised to an individual maximum on a bicycle ergometer according to the standard protocol of the cardiology department. Approximately 74 MBq (2 m Ci) was Tl 201 were injected at peak exercise, and the patient was asked to continue for 2 min more. Immediately after the exercise the patients were transferred to one of the SPECT instruments, and imaging commenced approximately 3 min later. Thereafter, 3 h were allowed for redistribution to occur and the patients were imaged again.

After PTCA the nuclear study was repeated, with patients exercising to the same level as before and using identical imaging parameters.

Evaluation

Each SPECT study, exercise period, and redistribution was examined for defects or decreased uptake of Tl 201. A finding was stated if a defect was present in two contiguous slices in two of the three reconstructed planes. The findings in the exercise study were compared with those of the same location in the redistribution study presenting (a) a persisting defect (pDEF) indicating severe ischemia and/or scar tissue, (b) a redistribution

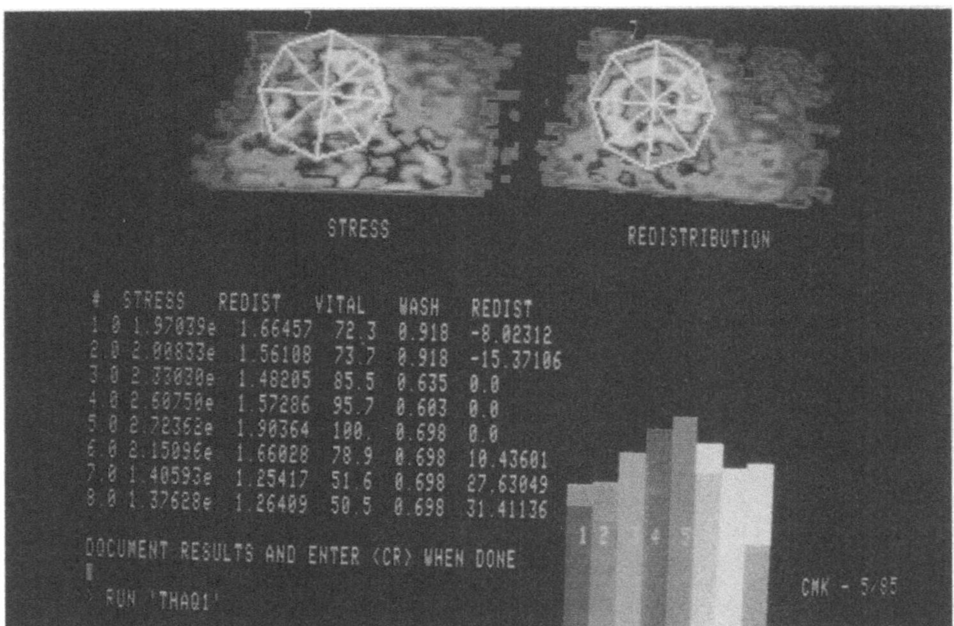

Fig. 1. Quantitative evaluation of the Tl 201 SPECT study before second PTCA (see also Fig. 7), with average VI of 60% and RDF of 23% in sectors 6-8 (anterior wall)

124

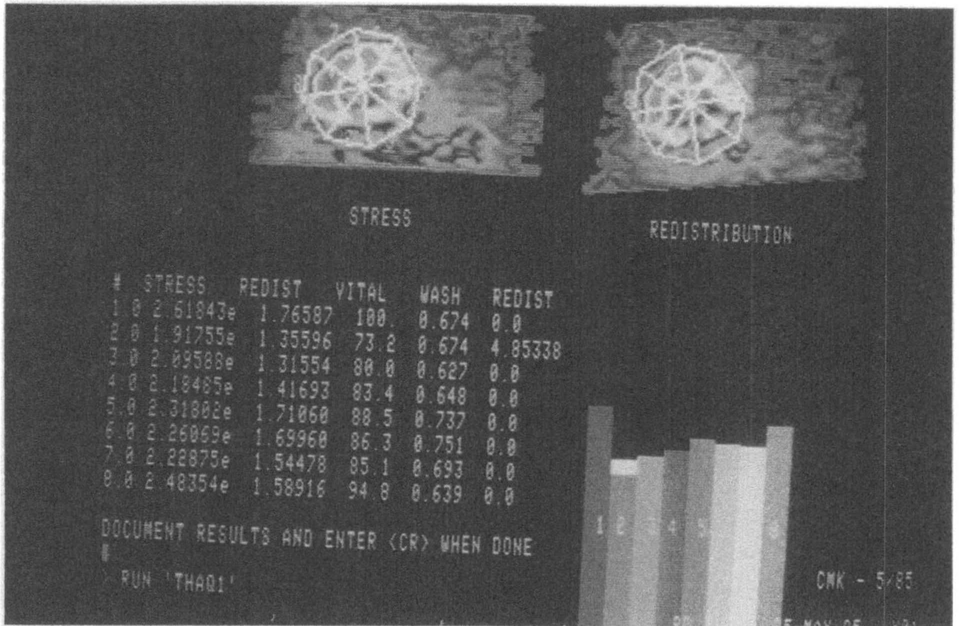

Fig. 2. After second PTCA (see also Fig. 7) average VI increased to 89% and RDF dropped to O; only marginal redistribution of 5% in sector 2 (inferior portion of the posterior wall)

pattern (RED), i.e., transient ischemia, or (c) a normal uptake. The location of the finding was reported, separating the anatomical structures into septum, anterior wall with an anterior and supra-apical portion, apex, lateral wall, and posterior wall with an inferior and posterior portion.

For the statistical evaluation two segments were defined: an anterior one comprising septum, anterior wall, apex, and the anterior parts of the lateral wall and a posterior one with the posterior wall and the posterior portion of the lateral wall.

For a quantitative evaluation of the SPECT studies a program was developed for the computer system connected to the ROTA camera [8, 9]. For quantification the exercise and redistribution slices of identical orientation and plane were selected under visual control. Eight congruent sectoral regions of interest were established over the myocardium (Figs. 1, 2) in each slice. Using the regional data the following parameters were calculated for each region: (a) a "viability index (VI)", defined as the ratio of the regional to the maximum uptake in the exercise study.

$$VI_I = \frac{CTS_{I\,EX}}{CTS_{MAX\,EX}} \cdot 100 \ [\%] \tag{1}$$

(b) a "wash-out factor (WO)" as the ratio of the regional count rate in the redistribution image to the one in the exercise image.

$$WF_I = \frac{CTS_{I\,Rest}}{CTS_{I\,EX}} \tag{2}$$

125

and (c) a "redistribution factor (RDF)" according to Eg. (3)

$$RDF_I = \frac{CTS_{I\,Rest}/WF_I - CTS_{I\,EX}}{CTS_{I\,EX}} \cdot 100 \, [\%] \tag{3}$$

For the statistical workup the average VIs and RDFs were formed in the slices before and after PTCA for neighboring sectors showing pathologic changes. Finally, the results of visual and quantitative evaluation were compared.

Results

Comparison of the segmental findings before and after PTCA showed the results given in Table 1. A total of 70 studies were performed and evaluated, since some patients presented restenosis with subsequent redilatation upon follow-up. Of the 15 segments that pre-

Table 1. Segmental findings before and after PTCA

Before		After PTCA		
	n	Norm	RED	pDEF
Norm	(64)	56	8	0
RED	(59)	43	15	1
pDEF	(17)	2	10	5
RED/RED (n = 15)		Improvement	8	
		No change	6	
		Deterioration	1	

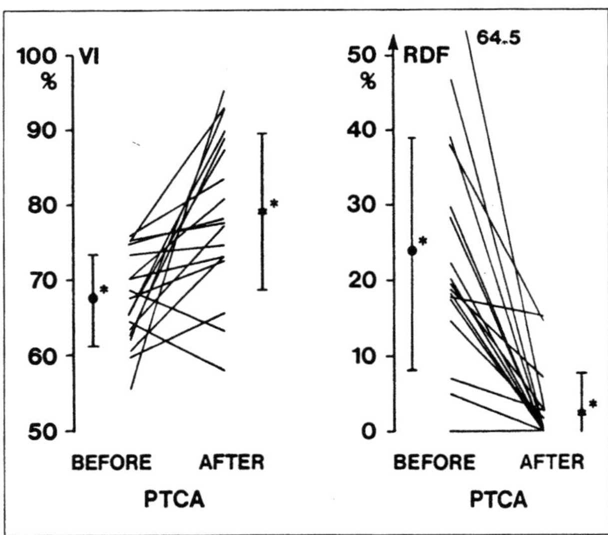

Fig. 3. Average VI and RDF before and after PTCA in 18 patients. Differences are significant (asterisks) for both factors (P < 0.001). VI was 67.3±5.8 before and 79.1±10.4 after; RDF was 23.6±15.2 before and 2.9±4.8 after PTCA

sented redistribution before and after PTCA, eight had improved, with a decrease of myocardium involved, six showed no change, and one showed deterioration. In addition, 18 studies of the 53 patients were evaluated quantitatively. A significant increase in the mean VI was found, as well as a significant reduction in RDF, as shown in Fig. 3.
Comparing the visual evaluation with the quantitative one for these 18 patients, we found agreement in five cases. In 13 cases the quantitative evaluation showed some remaining redistribution where none was detected visually.

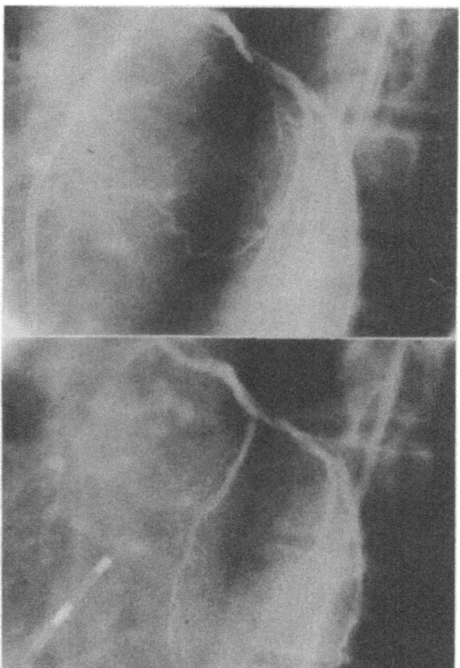

Fig. 4. Coronary angiogram of a 58-year-old patient with a high-grade stenosis of the LAD before **(upper)** and after **(lower)** first PTCA

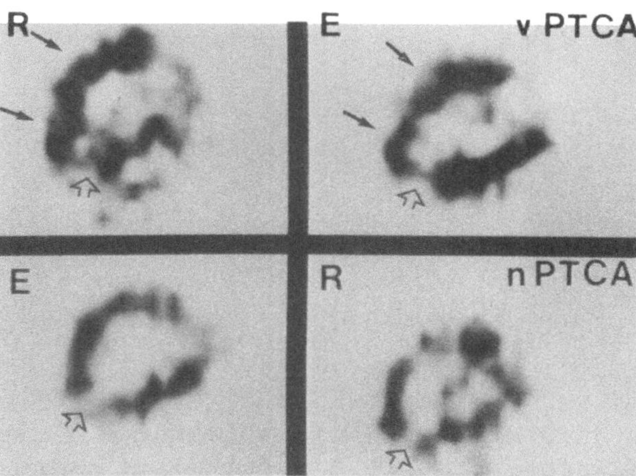

Fig. 5. Sagittal slice of the Tl 201 exercise (E)/redistribution (R) SPECT study before **(upper)** first PTCA, showing redistribution in the anterior wall **(arrow)** and a small persisting defect **(hollow arrow)** in the apex due to a previous MI. After PICA **(lower)** small apical defect remains but no redistribution

The clinical course of a 58-year-old male patient may serve as an example. When first seen, the patient complained of angina with a history of a small myocardial infarction in the anterior wall. Coronary angiography revealed a high-grade stenosis of the LAD, as shown in Fig. 4. The sagittal slices of the nuclear study (Fig. 5) showed marked redistribution in the anterior wall and a small apical defect before PTCA. After dilatation (Fig. 5, lower row) no transient ischemia could be identified, but the small apical defect due to the previous MI persisted. Upon follow-up 3 months later the patient had only minor discomfort when exercising. Angiography, however, revealed a recurrent stenosis of the LAD (Fig. 6, upper angiogram), and the repeated Tl 201 SPECT study (Fig. 7, upper row) presented redistribution in the anterior wall. After redilatation (Fig. 6, lower angiogram) the redistribution had disappeared (Fig. 7, lower row); only the small apical defect remained on visual evaluation.

The quantitative assessment before the second dilatation (Fig. 1) presented an average VI of 60% and an RDF of 23% for sectors 6-8 (anterior wall). After PTCA the average VI increased to 89% and the RDF dropped to zero (Fig. 2). Only a marginal redistribution (RDF = 5%) remained in sector 2 (inferior portion of the posterior wall).

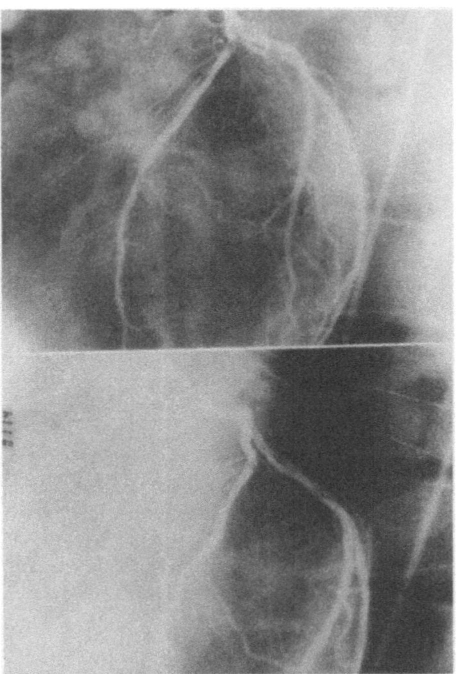

Fig. 6. Coronary angiogram of the same patient 3 months later with restenosis before (**upper**) and after (**lower**) second PTCA

Conclusions

Our recent experience shows that Tl 201 SPECT of the myocardium provides an excellent means for following up therapy. The success of PTCA can be monitored in terms of

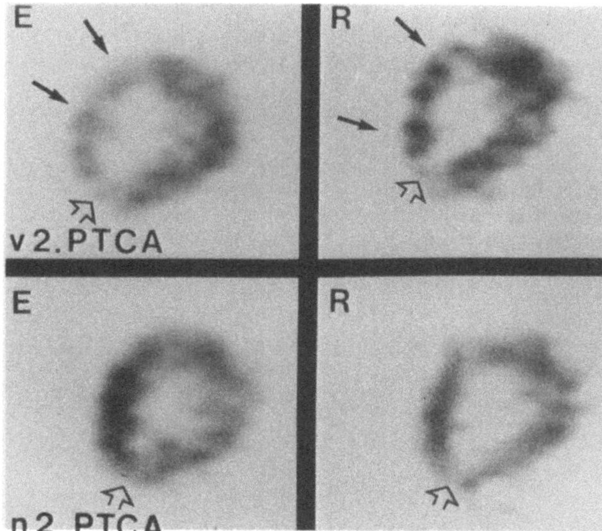

Fig. 7. Repeated Tl 201 SPECT study before **(upper)** second PTCA shows redistribution in the anterior wall **(arrows)** and the small apical defect **(hollow arrow)**; after **(lower)** PTCA no more redistribution. Quantitative evaluation see Fig. 1 und 2

myocardial viability and/or perfusion, as shown by the improvement in 50 of 58 segments (86%) with redistribution and 12 of 17 (70%) with a persisting defect. Applying a quantitative evaluation, the ischemia as well as the success of therapy can be graduated by the "viability index" and the "redistribution factor". Compared with a mere visual evaluation assessing only redistribution and/or a persisting defect, the VI is introduced as a further parameter.

As indicated by the possible improvement, persisting defects do not always represent scar tissue; they may also be due to severe ischemia. This finding can have major implications for the decision to perform PTCA.

References

1. Hoer G, Kannemoto N, (1981) 201-Tl myocardial scintigraphy: current status in coronary artery disease. Results of sensitivity/specificity in 3092 patients and clinical recommendations. Nucl Med 20:136
2. Kaltenbach M, Kober G, Scherer D, et al. (1981) Ergebnisse der transluminalen Koronarangioplastik. In: Breddin K (ed) Thrombose und Atherogenese, Pathophysiologie und Therapie der arteriellen Verschlußkrankheit, Bein-Beckenvenen-Thrombose. Witzstrock, Baden-Baden
3. Hoer G, Maul FD (1985) Beitrag der Myokardszintigraphie in der Therapiekontrolle (gegenwärtiger Stand und Ausblicke). Z Kardiol 74:65
4. Wijns W, Serruys PW, Reiber JHC et al. (1985) Early detection of restenosis after successful percutaneus transluminal coronary angioplasty by exercise-redistribution thallium scintigraphy. Am J Cardiol 55:357
5. Kirsch CM, Doliwa R, Buell U et al. (1983) Detection of severe coronary heart disease with Tl-201: comparison of resting single-photon-emission-tomography with invasive arteriography. J Nucl Med 24:761

6. Buell U, Doliwa R, Kirsch C-M et al. (1984) Die 201-Thallium-Single-Photon-Emissions-Computertomographie (SPECT) in der funktionellen Beurteilung koronarstenotischer Veränderungen. Ergebnisse des Vergleichs von belastungsszintigraphischen mit koronarangiographischen Befunden. Z Kardiol 73:313
7. Kirsch C-M, Doliwa R, Buell U, Höfling B (1985) Sensitivität und Spezifität von Belastungsuntersuchungen des Herzens mit Tl-201 in SPECT Technik. Der Nuklearmediziner 8/241
8. Kirsch C-M (1984) Numerische Gesichtspunkte bei der quantitativen Auswertung von Single-Photon-Emissions-Computertomographischen Studien (SPECT). NucCompact 15:316
9. Kirsch C-M, Moser E, Buell U (1986) Quantitative Auswertung von 201-Tl Myokardszintigrammen in SPECT Technik. NucCompact (in press)

Author's address:
Dr. med. Dipl.-Ing. Carl-Martin Kirsch
c/o Siemens Gammasonics Inc.
2000 Nuclear Drive
Des Plaines, IL 60018 USA

Is the candidate for PTCA always also a candiate for aortocoronary bypass operation?

H. C. Mehmel

II. Medizinische Klinik, Klinikum Karlsruhe

In its early days, PTCA was performed in patients with single-vessel disease, angina pectoris, and a pathologic exercise test, e.g., ST-segment depression, who were also considered for surgery at that time [1]. With increasing experience, skill, and development of the technique, patients with two- and three-vessel disease are now treated with PTCA, and for many of these patients an aortocoronary bypass operation is indicated as well. The question is whether every PTCA candidate should be also a candidate for surgery. In the early days of PTCA the answer was "yes". As the indications for surgery have become more restrictive in patients with mild angina pectoris, PTCA now is applied more frequently as an alternative to drug therapy rather than as an alternative to surgery.

At present, the general attitude is still to prefer PTCA for the patient with single-vessel disease and bypass surgery for the patient with multi-vessel disease (Fig. 1). This attitude is supported by the clinical follow-up of patients: with complete revascularization after PTCA, 80% of patients survive without symptoms or coronary events for 1 year, whereas with incomplete revascularization only 43% remain free of symptoms or coronary events. It is evident that the patient with single-vessel disease has the highest chance of complete revascularization after PTCA [2].

This attitude, on the other hand, means that PTCA will be recommended to a number of patients who are not considered candidates for surgery. A notable exception is the patient with a high-grade, proximal stenosis of the LAD without prior myocardial infarction. These patients usually have severe angina pectoris, which is poorly controlled by drug therapy, and they are good candidates for both PTCA and bypass surgery.

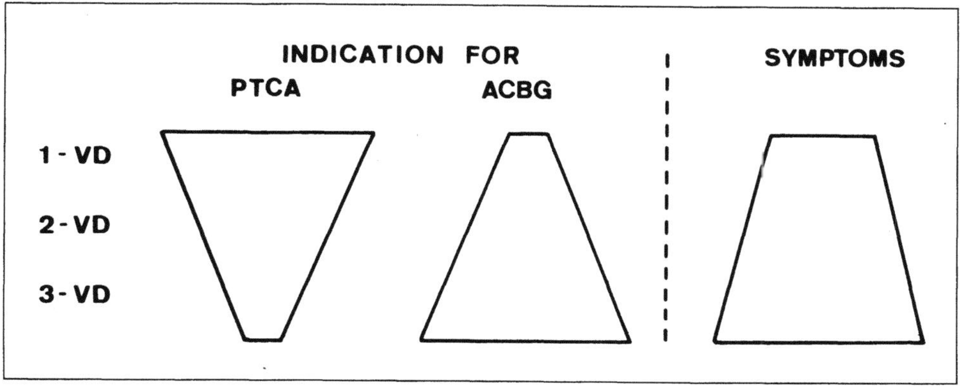

Fig. 1. Indications for percutaneous transluminal coronary angioplasty (PTCA) and aortocoronary bypass grafting (ACBG) in relation to the extent of coronary artery disease. 1-VD, single-vessel-disease; 2-VD, two-vessel disease; 3-VD, three-vessel disease

In most patients, however, symptoms usually correspond to the extent of the disease. It appears that PTCA is indeed viewed increasingly as an alternative to drug treatment rather than as an alternative to bypass surgery.

The complication rate, however, must be kept in mind; there is a fairly low mortality (2%) but a considerable overall complication rate (21%). In a study by the NHLBI the results of 3390 procedures at 105 sites are represented, i.e., an average of 34 patients per institution. The figures reported from individual centers with extensive experience are somewhat more favorable [3].

A considerable number (one third) of patients are operated on within the first few years after PTCA (33%), due partly to restenosis and partly to progression of the disease at other sites of the coronary artery tree [3].

Two special situations require brief comments:

1. Whereas PTCA may postpone coronary artery surgery, the situation is less favorable for PTCA after bypass surgery. The mortality of patients having native stenoses or graft stenoses dilated is unusually high. Probably these patients have more advanced disease. In addition, it takes longer to establish extracorporeal circulation in patients who have already been operated on. It appears, therefore, that the selection of patients for PTCA after bypass surgery must be done with extreme care.

2. In the patient with acute myocardial infarction, on the other hand, emergency PTCA, mostly in combination with thrombolysis, is preferable to emergency bypass surgery.

With respect to left ventricular function, aortocoronary bypass surgery appears to improve the prognosis in patients with three-vessel disease and with depressed left ventricular function, i.e., with a left ventricular ejection fraction in the range of 30%–50%. With regard to PTCA, the situation is not clarified. But most investigators in this field would probably agree that a compromised left ventricular function increases the risk of PTCA for the patient, e.g., for a patient with prior inferior myocardial infarction and a high-grade LAD stenosis. Any complication due to PTCA would carry a much higher risk for such a patient than for one with good left ventricular function. The consideration of left ventricular function suggests that the ideal candidate for PTCA cannot necessarily be considered a candidate for bypass surgery (Fig. 2).

Although prospective studies on the effect of PTCA on prognosis are still lacking, it appears most likely that this treatment of patients with single- or two-vessel disease, who

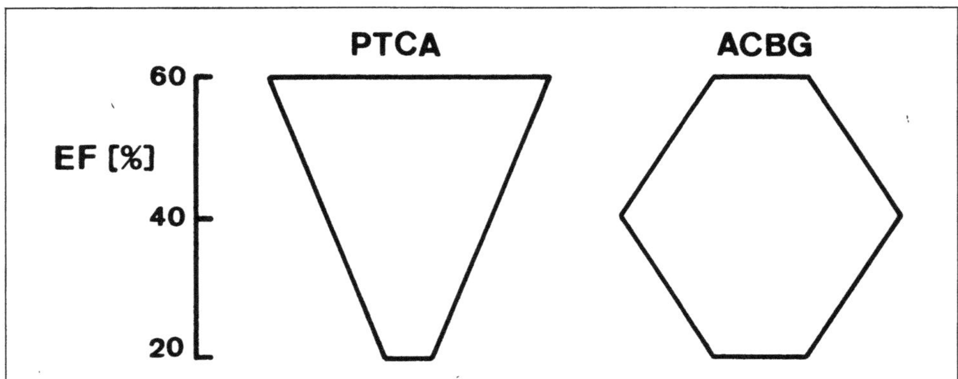

Fig. 2. Left ventricular function and indication for PTCA and ACBG. EF, ejection fraction

still represent the majority of patients considered for PTCA, will not improve prognosis, especially if one keeps the still fairly high recurrence rate in mind.

The recommendation to perform PTCA is therefore based predominantly on symptoms and/or pathologic exercise tests that are due to a circumscript and fairly localized distribution of coronary artery stenoses.

In summary, then, it appears, that there has been a kind of development from the early days of PTCA, when every candidate for PTCA was also a candidate for bypass surgery, to the attitude of today, when PTCA and bypass surgery are no longer competitive, but can be viewed as two procedures which may be offered to a patient in sequence as the disease progresses. In the future, however, the two interventions may become competitors again, when the technique of PTCA has progressed to such a degree that multi-vessel lesions can be treated by PTCA on a larger scale than is possible today (Fig. 3).

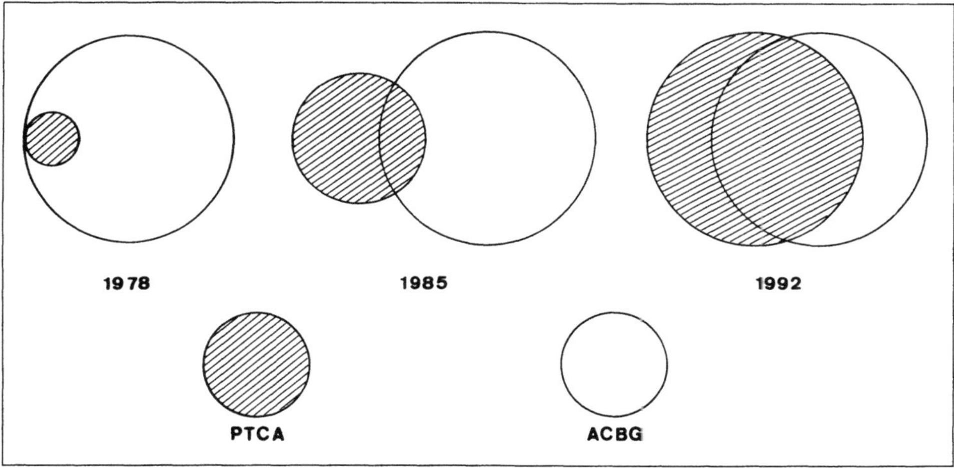

Fig. 3. Development of indications for PTCA and ACBG

References

1. Grüntzig A (1978) Transluminal dilatation of coronary artery stenosis. Lancet 1: 263
2. Meier B, Grüntzig AR, Siegenthaler WE, Schlumpf M (1983) Long-term exercise performance after percutaneous transluminal coronary angioplasty and coronary artery bypass grafting. Circulation 68: 796
3. Dorros G, Cowley MJ, Simpson J et al. (1983) Percutaneous transluminal coronary angioplasty: report of complications from the National Heart, Lung, and Blood Institute PTCA registry. Circulation 67: 723

Author's address:
Prof. Dr. H. C. Mehmel
Klinikum Karlsruhe
II. Medizinische Klinik
Moltkestraße 14
7500 Karlsruhe

Complementary Relationships of Coronary Bypass Surgery and Percutaneous Transluminal Coronary Angioplasty

J. S. Douglas, Jr.*

Andreas Gruentzig Cardiovascular Center, Emory University School of Medicine, Atlanta, Georgia USA

It is a rare patient whose immediate need for coronary revascularization requires simultaneous application of both coronary artery bypass grafting (CABG) and percutaneous transluminal coronary angioplasty (PTCA). Many patients, however, have required these two forms of therapy at different points in time, and there is an even greater number of patients who have had a revascularization procedure but, because of the progressive nature of the disease, will need a second procedure in the future. Excellence in both forms of therapy is now required to provide for the patient optimal revascularization results at the lowest monetary and morbidity costs.

It is only natural that proponents of each mode of myocardial revascularization (CABG and PTCA) will strive to achieve the most effective and long-lasting treatment possible. The complementary nature of these procedures is evident in many clinical circumstances.

Extremes of Age and Disease

PTCA offers to the young patient and the patient with focal coronary obstruction a less invasive revascularization alternative, preserving conduits and future surgical options. In progressive disease the need for reoperations with the attendant increased risk and cost is minimized.

In the aged, PTCA is an effective, low-risk procedure [1, 2] which can relieve surgical resources of the complications and longer convalescence which is characteristic of this population [3, 4]. PTCA is not best suited for severe diffuse proximal coronary disease where internal mammary artery grafting is the most effective therapy, yielding a high 7–10 year graft patency [5]. It is only proper that the severity of the treatment (risk, morbidity, and cost) should bear some relationship to the severity of the disease, and this tends to be true in the use of CABG and PTCA to treat obstructive coronary artery disease.

---

* Associate Professor of Medicine (Cardiology) and Assistant Professor of Radiology, Emory University School of Medicine. Co-Director of Cardiac Laboratories, Emory University Hospital

Contraindications

Many patients with severe coexistent medical problems such as pulmonary insufficiency, hematologic disorders, immunologic suppression, cancer, and renal insufficiency tolerate PTCA quite well, precluding the need for entanglements in complex and protracted postoperative complications encountered with coronary bypass grafting [6].

Occasionally, patients with contraindications to CABG, such as the absence of suitable conduits or inadequate left ventricular function, can be managed by PTCA. However, the lack of a means of surgical rescue in case of PTCA failure tempers our enthusiasm for this approach. Many patients with severe angina and even the poorest left ventricular function can be managed surgically with acceptable risk and good relief of symptoms [7].

Treatment Failures

Perhaps the most obvious complementary relationship between CABG and PTCA teams exists when failure of one mode of therapy can be compensated for by the other. Most often, the surgeon is called upon to "bail out" the angioplasty physician when acute coronary occlusion occurs post angioplasty, but surgeon and patient are genuinely grateful when the roles are reversed (Fig. 7).

PTCA Failure

Acute coronary occlusion post PTCA occurs in 3%–5% of patients, and although there are known factors associated with increased risk of occlusion (multivessel disease, length, eccentricity, tortuosity), acute occlusion remains unpredictable [8]. It appears that approximately 50% of acute closures can be satisfactorily managed with repeat angioplasty, and most persistent failures require emergency coronary bypass surgery. At Emory University Hospital, over 200 emergency operations for failed PTCA have been performed, with a 2% operative mortality. Although one half of the patients had evidence of acute myocardial infarction, less than a quarter had Q-wave infarctions. Six of seven patients taken to the operating room with sustained closed chest massage in progress were saved. All would have died without immediate surgery. The prompt availability of excellent emergency surgery minimizes risk in routine PTCA, and this support allows expansion of indications for PTCA to high-risk patients who would not otherwise be candidates. The risk of any PTCA is determined by the coronary anatomy and left ventricular function, but also by the quality of the surgical backup.

CABG Failure

Early failures of coronary bypass surgery which are amenable to PTCA include the presence of unbypassed vessels, graft thrombosis when the native coronary artery can be dilated, and perianastomotic stenosis of vein grafts or internal mammary arteries (Fig. 2) [9, 10]. Our experience indicates that a 95% long-term success rate can be achieved with PTCA of stenoses developing in the distal saphenous vein graft anastomosis within 6

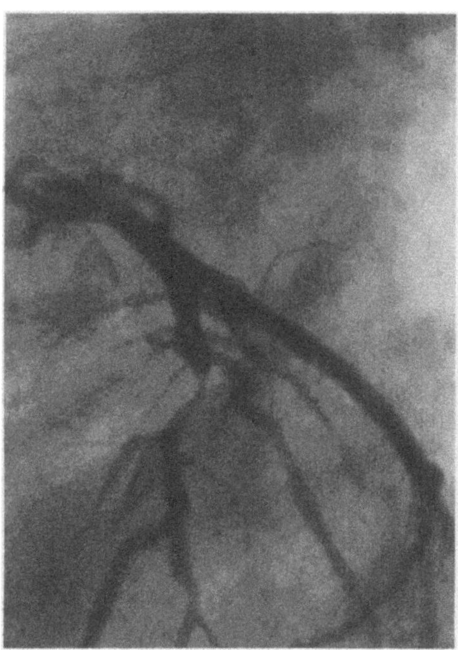

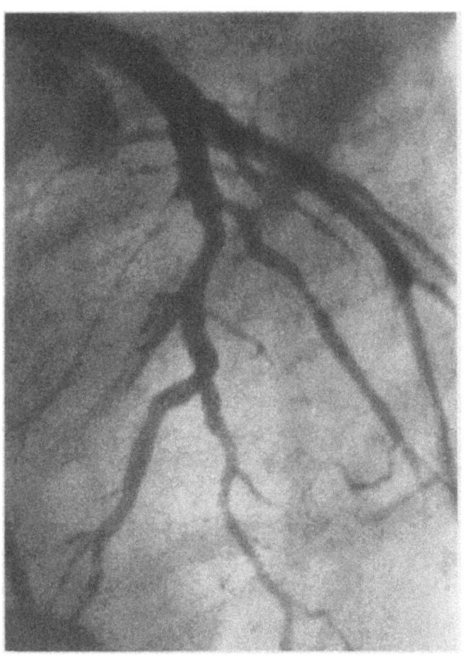

Fig. 1a, b. High-grade stenosis of the mid-left anterior descending coronary artery occurred during the first year following cardiac transplantation (a). PTCA was performed with excellent angiographic results (b), delaying need for reoperation.

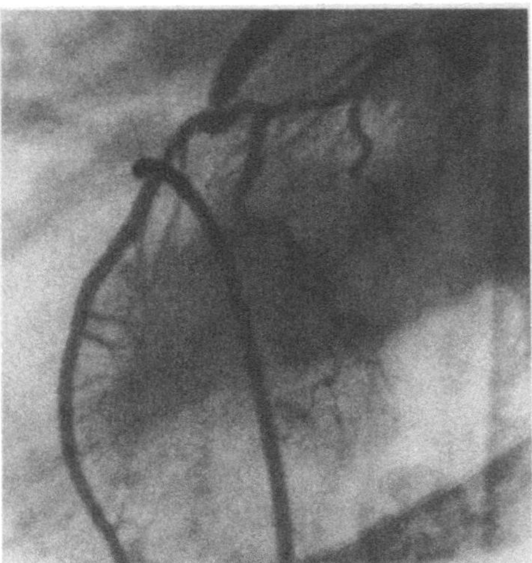

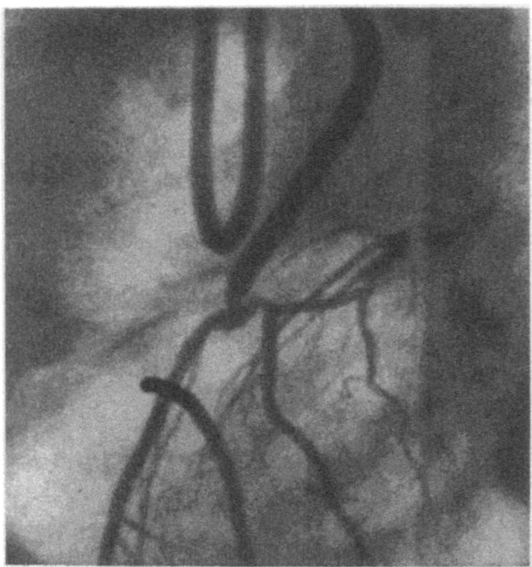

Fig. 2a, b. Saphenous vein graft implantation site stenosis (a) of the left anterior descending coronary graft was treated effectively with PTCA, producing a widely patent anastomosis (b) and relief of angina.

months of surgery (9, 10, 11). Early stenoses occurring in the mid portion of the vein graft have only a 50% long-term success rate; however, these stenoses can be treated with angioplasty at extremely low risk.

Late surgical failures occurring due to progression of disease in the vein grafts or native coronary arteries can frequently be managed with PTCA. Although stenoses of the proximal and mid portions of vein grafts have a high initial PTCA success rate, the recurrence rate is also high, yielding less than 50% long-term success (Fig. 3). In addition, in vein grafts implanted for over 3 years, 3%–5% of carefully selected cases in our experience have evidence of vein graft atheroemboli at the time of PTCA, resulting in myocardial infarction [12].

138

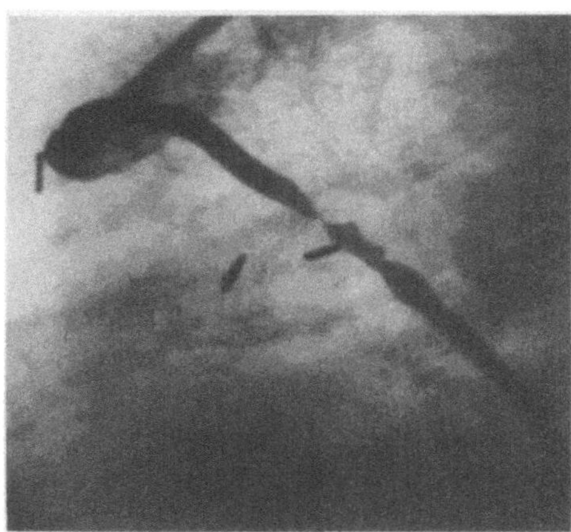

Fig. 3a–c. Unstable angina was relieved by successful PTCA of a stenosis in the mid portion of a saphenous vein graft to the circumflex coronary artery implanted for 7 years. The initial success rate for this lesion should exceed 95%, and coronary embolization is rare [12]. Restenosis, however, is common [11]. High grade stenosis (a); balloon inflation to 10 atms (b), resulted in widely patent conduit (c)

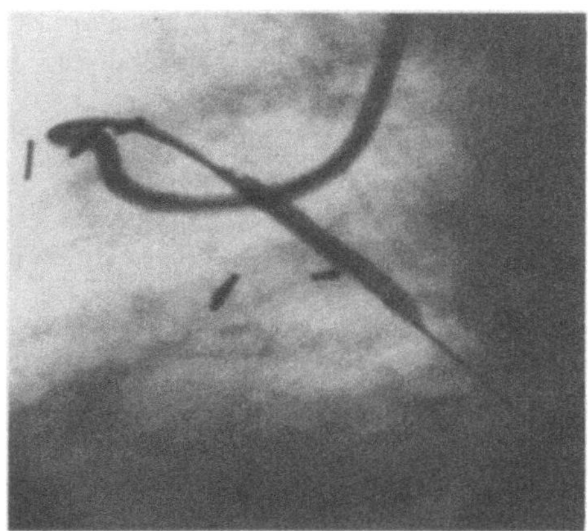

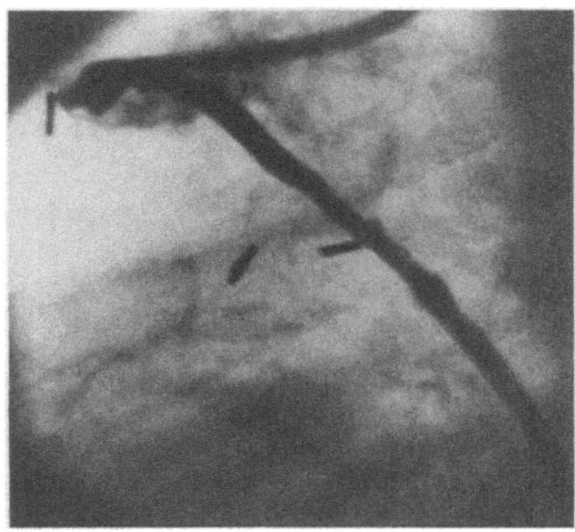

In general, selection of post CABG patients for PTCA must be done with great care, since surgical reinstitution of coronary flow following failed PTCA is substantially delayed due to the technical problems involved in reoperative surgery. No deaths, however, have occurred at Emory University Hospital in over 600 elective PTCA procedures in patients with prior bypass surgery. This can be contrasted with the 3%–9% reported mortality for reoperation by experienced surgeons [13–15].

Acute Myocardial Infarction

Although it is clear that emergency coronary bypass surgery is effective therapy for acute myocardial infarction [16], the logistic problems and the expense of providing this therapy are prohibitive. Thrombolytic therapy and PTCA have moved to the forefront in treatment of acute myocardial infarction, relieving surgical teams of this responsibility, and by preserving myocardial function these methods retain for many patients with multivessel disease the option of elective CABG. Some patients, however, still require emergency bypass surgery for repeated closure at the PTCA site when it is clear that myocardial salvage has taken place. The need for close interrelation of the angioplasty and surgical teams in planning surgery for recanalized patients with multivessel disease is apparent.
The roles of PTCA and CABG are evolving as experience, new technology, and new insights are acquired. The angioplasty physician and the surgeon must continue to work together to achieve for the patient the optimal revascularization possible at the lowest risk and monetary cost. Only then can the complementary relationship of these different procedures be fully explored.

References

1. Abi-Mansour P, Roubin G, Rice C, Bredlau C, Douglas J, King S, Gruentzig A (1986) Restenosis and late cardiac events after successful coronary angioplasty in elderly patients. J Am Coll Cardiol 7 (2): 19A
2. Mock MB, Holmes DR Jr., Vlietstra RE, Gersh BJ, Detre KM, Kelsey SF, et al. (1984) Percutaneous transluminal coronary angioplasty in the elderly patient: experience in the National Heart, Lung, and Blood Institute PTCA Registry. Am J Cardiol 53: 89C–91C
3. Knapp WS, Douglas JS jr, Craver JM, Jones EL, King SB III, Bone DK, Bradford JM, Hatcher CR (1981) Efficacy of coronary artery bypass grafting in elderly patients with coronary artery disease. Am J Cardiol 47: 923–930
4. Gann D, Cohn C, Hildner FJ, Samet P, Yahr WZ, Greenberg JJ (1977) Coronary artery bypass surgery in patients seventy years of age and older. J Thorac Cardiovasc Surg 73: 237–241
5. Lytle BW, Loop FD, Cosgrove DM, Ratliff NB, Easley K, Taylor PC (1985) Long-term (5–12 years) serial studies of internal mammary artery and saphenous vein coronary bypass grafts. J Thorac Cardiovasc Surg 89: 248–258
6. Taylor GJ, Rabinovich E, Mikell FL, Moses HW, Dove JT, Batchelder JE, Wellons HA jr., Schneider JA (1986) Percutaneous transluminal coronary angioplasty as palliation for patients considered poor surgical candidates. Am Heart J 111: 840–844
7. Jones EL, Craver JM, Kaplan JA, et al. (1978) Criteria for operability and reduction of surgical mortality in patients with severe left ventricular ischemia and dysfunction. Ann Thorac Surg 25 (5): 413–424
8. Bredlau C, Roubin G, Leimgruber P, Douglas J, King S, Gruentzig A (1985) In-hospital morbidity and mortality in elective coronary angioplasty. Circulation 72: 1044–1052

9. Douglas JS, Gruentzig AR, King SB, Hollman J et al. (1983) Percutaneous transluminal coronary angioplasty in patients with prior coronary bypass surgery. J Am Coll Cardiol 2 (4): 745–754
10. Zaidi AR, Hollman JL (1985) Percutaneous angioplasty of internal mammary artery graft stenosis: case report and discussion. Cathet Cardiovasc Diagn 11: 603–608
11. Douglas J, King S, Roubin G, Schlumpf, M (1986) Percutaneous angioplasty of venous aortocoronary graft stenoses: late angiographic and clinical outcome. Circulation 74 (Supp II): II, 281
12. Douglas J, King S, Roubin G, Schlumpf M (1986) Percutaneous transluminal angioplasty in aortocoronary venous graft stenoses: immediate results and complications. Circulation 74 (Supp II): II, 363
13. Hall RB, Elayfda MA, Gray AG, Cooley DA (1986) Reoperation for coronary artery disease. J Am Coll Cardiol 7 (2): 32A
14. Brenowitz J, Dorros G, Schley L, Johnson WD (1986) Coronary artery bypass graft surgery for the third time or more. The results of 90 consecutive operations. J Am Coll Cardiol 7(2): 31A
15. Lytle BW, Loop FD, Cosgrove DM, Taylor PC, et al (1986) Fifteen hundred coronary reoperations: results and determinants of early and late survival. J Am Coll Cardiol 7(2): 31A
16. Berg JR, Selinger SL, Leonard JJ, Grunwald RP, O'Grady WP (1981) Immediate coronary artery bypass for acute evolving myocardial infarction. J Thorac Cardiovasc Surg 81: 493–497

Author's address:
John S. Douglas, Jr., M.D.
Emory University Hospital
Cardiac Cath Lab
1364 Clifton Rd. N.E.
Atlanta, Georgia 30322, USA
(404) 727–7034

Surgical Procedures During Evolving Infarction and After Thrombolysis and Unsuccessful PTCA

B. Reichart

Department of Cardiac-Thoracis Surgery, Groote-Schuus Hospitel, Red Cross Children's Hospital, Medical School, University of Cape Town

Experimental and Clinical Background

It was originally believed that the fate of an ischemic myocardium was determined within 60 min. In 1975, however, Constantini et al. [1] demonstrated in animal experiments that revascularization after 3 h of LAD occlusion significantly reduced the expected average infarct size. Cardiac metabolism remained abnormal or deteriorated further for at least 1 h after reperfusion but returned to normal after a week. Restoration of cardiac function usually also occurred by the 7th day. These findings were confirmed by Maroko et al. [2] in short-term reperfusion experiments.

These two studies showed that, in general, the full extent of the myocardial necrosis does not occur until 3 h have elapsed. Within this period the ischemic tissue may be salvageable, though the extent of necrosis and the rapidity with which it occurs depend on both the coronary artery collateral flow and myocardial oxygen requirements.

As the above-mentioned experimental work was performed in normal dogs, one would expect that the 3-h limit could be extended in human beings with long-standing atheromatous heart disease who may have developed increased collateral flow.

In the early 1970s, Dawson et al. [3] published data on aortocoronary artery bypass surgery in human beings performed "early" after acute myocardial infarction. When the revascularization took place within 24 h, the operative mortality of 44% was discouragingly high. Mortality remained high when revascularization was performed within 2 or 7 days (33% and 43% respectively). It should be noted that most of these patients had a complicated postinfarction course with symptoms of cardiogenic shock, requiring repeated cardiac resuscitation. In general, death occurred in the operating room; complete transmural infarction must therefore be assumed.

The study of Dawson et al. belongs to the pre-cardioplegia era; more recently, Hochberg et al. [4] repeated the survey, using potassium cardioplegia to protect the myocardium during surgery. Yet the initial mortality was again high (46% and 33% respectively) when surgery was accomplished within the first 1 or 2 weeks in patients with postinfarct ejection fractions equal to or below 50%. (No patient was lost whose ejection fraction was greater than 50%.) When revascularization was performed 4–5 weeks after the day of infarction, survival rates steadily improved. Patients with a low postinfarct ejection fraction, however, continued to show a higher long-term mortality – the 5- to 6-year survival rate was 97% in the group with a normal ejection fraction, but it decreased to 65% in patiens with low values.

Summarizing these more recent clinical data, one can conclude that, to obtain good results, revascularization after acute myocardial infarction should obviously be performed very early, within a few hours, or very late, after more than 4–5 weeks.

Emergency Aortocoronary Bypass Surgery

The first to demonstrate that early revascularization (in the true sense of Constantini and Maroko) was feasible were Loop et al. from the Cleveland Clinic in 1975 [5]. In about two thirds of their 37 patients, the acute event was initiated in the catheterization laboratory of the cardiologists. All patients were revascularized within 6 h, and the early mortality was only 14%.

Berg's group from Spokane [6] performed early revascularization in patients who were referred with signs of an evolving myocardial infarction. The following features were considered to be significant: on-going chest pain, new Q waves longer than 0.04 s in duration, ST injury pattern, major (more than 90%) coronary artery lesions or left ventricular abnormalities on angiography (which was completed on average within 35 min), and massively elevated enzyme levels (though peak values occurred after surgery).

The decision whether to treat a patient surgically or medically was shared with the cardiologist. Those selected for emergency coronary artery bypass surgery were patients who were less than 6 h in the infarction syndrome and who had evolving infarction due to stenosis or occlusion of dominant vessels – mainly the LAD (Fig. 1). No patient was turned down for surgery because of age, arrhythmias, pulmonary edema, or cardiogenic shock.

Two hundred and forty-one patients were operated on; the early and late death rates were 2.3% and 1.2% respectively, and the subsequent quality of life was claimed to improve in 95.9% of the cases.

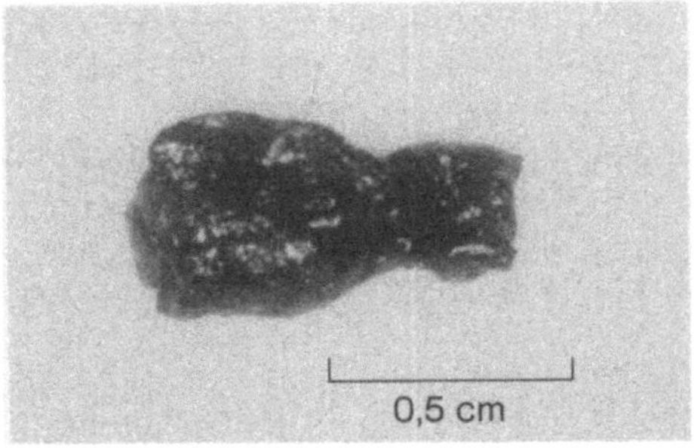

Fig. 1. Fresh clot removed from the LAD

Phillips et al. [7] reported on a group of 181 patients suffering from evolving myocardial infarction; the early surgical mortality was reported to be 5.5%. In contrast to Berg's group, Phillips and his colleagues did not believe in a strict time limit of 6 h. Some of their interventions were completed as late as 36 h after the onset of features suggesting evolving infarction, the average being approximately 8 h. Rather, they described two factors which, in their hands, proved beneficial in regard to successful revascularization:

Early surgery was indicated whenever on-going ischemic chest pain existed, on condition that the endocardium of the threatened area remained normal in appearance on angiography, being smooth and lightly trabeculated. On the other hand, surgery appeared to be contra-indicated when the endocardial surface appeared irregular, mottled, or fingerprinted, or contained filling defects; in these cases, regions were assumed to have undergone advanced myocardial necrosis.

Thrombolysis with Streptokinase

In recent times, emergency revascularization as a form of therapy during evolving myocardial infarction has been successfully challenged by intracoronary streptokinase thrombolysis. In the near future the efficacy of simple intravenous streptokinase therapy [8] will
become clearer, as will that of the more sophisticated tissue plasminogen activator [9]
and thromboxane synthetase inhibitors [10].

Since the early reocclusion rate following streptokinase treatment is in the area of 40% –
depending on the geometry of the residual coronary artery lesion [11] – thrombolysis has
been combined with either PTCA or, in cases with more diffuse coronary artery disease,
surgical revascularization (Fig. 2). The question which remains, and which is under de-
bate today, is the exact timing of the intervention. Since early surgery seems to carry an
increased risk with regard to the complication rate and the mortality [7, 12], it is now
generally agreed that the patient first be allowed to "cool off" and overcome the acute
phase of the myocardial infarction. Revascularization may then be undertaken within a
week at a low risk, with a mortality reported to be between 0 and 2% [13-16].

PTCA and Evolving Infarction

Failure of PTCA may occur either early after the procedure or late. Early failure of
PTCA is defined whenever the obstruction in the coroary artery cannot be reached or
crossed with the balloon catheter or when the gradient of the stenosis remains unchanged.

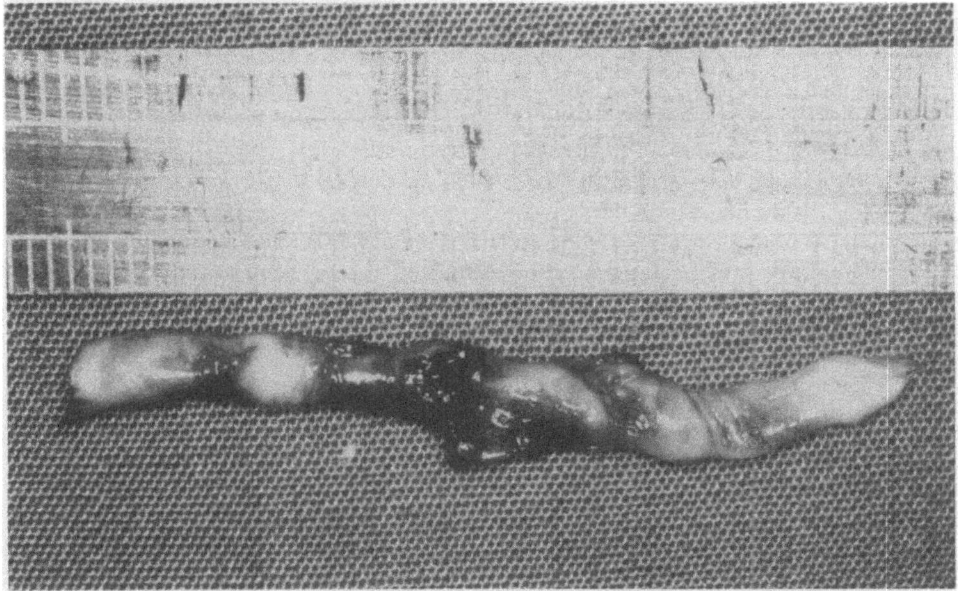

Fig. 2. Endarterectomy of an arteriosclerotic plaque which was located in the right coronary artery; the
plaque is opened up and reveals a fresh thrombus

Emergency revascularization is indicated in early failure only when features of acute myocardial ischemia are present, such as protracted chest pain, ECG changes, and clinical symptoms of decreased cardiac output. If possible, angiography should be attempted in order to establish the exact pathology of the lesions.

According to the American National Heart, Lung and Blood Institute registry, emergency surgery after PTCA was necessary in 203 (6.6%) of 3079 cases [17]. The indication for operation was coronary artery dissection in 46.6% of the cases, coronary artery occlusion in 20%, prolonged angina in 14%, and coronary artery spasm in 11%. No absolute clinical features predicting that emergency surgery might be required could be identified; however, eccentric lesions were more likely to be associated with complications. The need for emergency revascularization declined as the experience of the cardiologist with this procedure increased.

Akins and Block [18] noted that complications of PTCA occurred more commonly in women than in men (14.7% versus 6.6%), and also in patients with right coronary artery lesions. These observations may be explained by the smaller vessel size in women and by the anatomy of the right coronary artery, which changes direction sharply 1-2 cm distal to its orifice.

During a 10 month survey, 17 patients at Emory University in Atlanta needed emergency revascularization, a procedure which was carried out in the first operating room that became available. There were no deaths related to surgery [19].

The indications for revascularization were severe chest pain and ST-segment elevation on the ECG. Though the time from onset of ischemia to revascularization averaged only 135 min, 71% (12 patients) experienced complete transmural infarction, as did all who demonstrated ST-segment elevation. The development of myocardial necrosis did not correlate with the time which had elapsed between the event and successful reperfusion of the jeopardized area, or with the number of diseased vessels, the type of artery damaged, the mechanism of ischemia, or the presence of collateral flow.

Therefore, a high proportion of the patients who experienced coronary artery injury after PTCA tended to develop irreversible transmural necrosis rather quickly. Since, under these circumstances, the time between the onset of ischemia and successful revascularization is obviously too long, Murphy et al. recommended the immediate introduction of intra-aortic balloon counterpulsation [20]. They claimed that with the help of this circulatory assist device the infarction rate was reduced to 30%.

Reviewing the literature and summing up our own experience, it becomes difficult to provide an incontrovertible recommendation as to how to proceed in emergency cases after PTCA has failed (a situation which undoubtedly puts a great deal of psychological pressure on the dilating cardiologist). In view of the low mortality related to surgery, we would suggest surgery in cases which are complicated by a dissected major coronary artery, such as the LAD or a dominant right coronary artery. Prolonged ischemic chest pain requiring morphine would be an additional factor suggesting an emergency intervention was indicated.

In recent times, the indication for surgery has been questioned whenever an occlusion of the coronary artery has been diagnosed. While Schofer et al. [21] favored reopening by intracoronary streptokinase, Hollman et al. [22] recommended treatment with nitrates and calcium antagonists, or even repeat angioplasty. Whenever acute occlusion had been successfully resolved, patients were stabilized on a continuous i.v. infusion of nitroglycerine and heparin.

146

To summarize with a look to the future, PTCA seems to be a safe technique with a low complication rate; the necessity for emergency aortocoronary bypass surgery should be expected to be between 3% and 4%. On the other hand, the need for PTCA may still increase; PTCA has been used successfully in addition to a cardiosurgical procedure – either in the operating room during revascularization, when distal or inaccessible proximal lesions were dilated [23], or in the late postoperative course, when stenosed saphenous vein grafts have required dilatation [24, 25]. Only recently, a cardiac transplant patient suffering from chronic rejection was reported to have undergone successful coronary artery dilatation [26].

PTCA and aortocoronary artery bypass surgery are not rival techniques – on the contrary, they complement each other in the long-term treatment of patients suffering from severe coronary artery disease.

References

1. Constantini, C., Corday E, Lang TW, Meerbaum S, Brasch J, Kaplan J, Rubin S, Gold H, Osher J (1975) Revascularization after 3 hours of coronary arterial occlusion. Effects on regional cardiac metabolic function and infarct size. Am J Cardiol 36: 368
2. Maroko PR, Quinks WR, Libby P, Sobel BE, Shell WE, Ross J (1973) Salvage of myocardial tissue by coronary artery reperfusion following acute coronary occlusion. Am J Cardiol 2: 278
3. Dawson JT, Hall RJ, Hallman GL, Cooley DA (1974) Mortality in patients undergoing coronary artery bypass surgery after myocardial infarction. Am J Cardiol 33: 483
4. Hochberg MS, Parsonnet V, Gielchinsky J, Hussein SM, Fisch DA, Norman JC (1984) Timing of coronary revascularization after acute myocardial infarction. J Thorac Cardiovasc Surg 88: 914
5. Loop FD, Cheanvechai C, Sheldon WC, Taylor PC, Effleo DE (1974) Early myocardial revascularization during acute myocardial infarction. Chest 66: 478
6. Berg R, Selinger SL, Leonard JJ, Grunwald RP, Grady WP (1982) Surgical management of acute myocardial infarction. In: McGoon DC (ed) Cardiac surgery, p 61
7. Phillips SJ, Kongtahworn C, Skinner JR, Zeff RH, Dorner RA (1983) Emergency coronary artery reperfusion. A choice therapy for evolving myocardial infarction. J Thorac Cardiovasc Surg 86: 679
8. Losman JG, Newell R, Nagle D, Dacumos GC, Jones CR, Wilensky AS, Martin RG, Bailey MT, Kahn DR (1985) Myocardial surgical revascularization after streptokinase treatment for acute myocardial infarction. J Thorac Cardiovasc Surg 89: 25
9. Soebel BE, Gelfman EM, Trefenbrunn AJ, Jaffe AS, Spadaro JJ, Ter-Pogossian MM, Collen D, Ludbrook PA (1984) Improvement of regional myocardial metabolism after coronary thrombolysis induced with tissue-type plasminogen activator or streptokinase. Circulation 69: 983
10. Bush LR, Campbell WB, Buja M, Tilton G, Willerson JT (1984) Effects of the selective thromboxane synthetase inhibitor dazoxiben on variations in cyclic blood flow in stenosed canine coronary arteries. Circulation 69: 1161
11. Harrison DG, Ferguson DW, Collins SM, Skorton DJ, Ericksen EE, Kioschos JM, Marcus ML, White CW (1984) Rethrombosis after reperfusion with streptokinase: importance of geometry of residual lesions. Circulation 69: 991
12. Skinner JR, Phillips SJ, Zeff RH, Kongtahworn C (1984) Immediate coronary bypass following failed streptokinase infusion in evolving myocardial infarction. J Thorac Cardiovasc Surg 27: 567
13. Messmer BJ, Merx W, Meyer J, Bardos P, Minale C, Effert S (1983) New developments in medical-surgical treatment of acute myocardial infarction. Ann Thorac Surg 35: 70
14. Wilson JM, Held JS, Wright CB, Abbottsmith CW, Callard GM, Mitts DL, Dunn EJ, Melvil DB, Flege JB (1984) Coronary artery bypass surgery following thrombolytic therapy for acute coronary thrombosis. Ann Thorac Surg 37: 212

15. Krebber HJ, Schofer J, Mathey D, Moutz R, Kalmar P, Rodewald G, Hill JD (1984) Intracoronary thallium-201 scintigraphy as an immediate predictor of salvaged myocardium following intracoronary lysis. J Thorac Cardiovasc Surg 87: 27
16. Sterling RP, Walker WE, Weiland AP, Freund GC, Fuentes F, Smalling RW, Gould KL (1984) Early bypass grafting following intracoronary thrombolysis with streptokinase. J Thorac Cardiovasc Surg 87: 487
17. Cowley MJ, Dorros G, Kelsey SL, van Raden M, Detre KM (1984) Emergency coronary bypass surgery after coronary angioplasty: The National Heart, Lung and Blood Institute's percutaneous transluminal coronary angioplasty registry experience. Am J Cardiol 53: 22C
18. Akins CW, Block PC (1984) Surgical intervention for failed percutaneous transluminal coronary angioplasty. Am J Cardiol 53: 108C
19. Murphy DA, Craver JM, Jones EL, Grüntzig AR, King SB, Hatcher CR (1982) Surgical revascularization following unsuccessful percutaneous transluminal coronary angioplasty. J Thorac Cardiovasc Surg 84: 342
20. Murphy DA, Craver JM, Jones EL, Curling PE, Guyton RA, King SB, Grüntig AR, Hatcher CR (1984) Surgical management of acute myocardial ischemia following percutaneous transluminal coronary angioplasty. J Thorac Cardiovasc Surg 87: 332
21. Schofer J, Krebber HJ, Bleifeld W, Mathey DG (1982) Acute coronary artery occlusion during percutaneous transluminal coronary angioplasty: reopening by intracoronary streptokinase before emergency coronary artery surgery to prevent myocardial infarction. Circulation 66: 1325
22. Hollman J, Grüntzig AR, Douglas JS, King SB, Ischinger T, Meier B (1983) Acute occlusion after percutaneous transluminal coronary angioplasty – a new approach. Circulation 68: 725
23. Roberts AJ, Faro RS, Feldman RL, Conti CR, Knauf DG, Alexander JA, Pepine CJ (1983) Comparison of early and long-term results with intraoperative transluminal balloon catheter dilatation and coronary artery bypass grafting. J Thorac Cardiovasc Surg 86: 435
24. Jones EL, Douglas JS, Grüntzig AR, Craver JM, King SB, Guyton RA, Hatcher CR (1983) Percutaneous saphenous vein angioplasty to avoid reoperative bypass surgery. Ann Thorac Surg 36: 389
25. Dorros G, Johnson WD, Tector AJ, Schmahl TM, Kabush SL, Janke L (1984) Percutaneous transluminal coronary angioplasty in patients with prior coronary bypass grafting. J Thorac Cardiovasc Surg 87: 17
26. Hastillo A, Cowley MJ, Vetrovec G, Wolfgang TC, Lower RR, Hess ML (1985) Serial coronary angioplasty for arteriosclerosis following heart transplantation. Heart Transplantation 4: 192

Author's address:
Prof. Dr. B. Reichart
Department of Cardio-Thoracic Surgery
Medical School
Observatory
7925 Cape Town
South Africa